LOW OXALATE FOOD LIST

The Do's and Don'ts

Claudia Adkins

LEGAL DISCLAIMER

This book serves as educational and entertainment material and is not a substitute for professional medical advice or treatment. While the information presented here is sourced from reliable outlets to the best of the Author's knowledge, accuracy cannot be guaranteed. The Author cannot be held responsible for any errors or omissions. It is advisable to consult a medical professional before implementing any remedies or techniques suggested in this book.

By utilizing the information provided, you agree to absolve the Author and Publisher of any liability for damages, expenses, or legal fees arising from the application of the advice contained herein. This disclaimer encompasses any damages or injuries resulting directly or indirectly from the use of the information presented, regardless of the cause of action.

You acknowledge and assume all risks associated with the utilization of the information within this book. It is recommended to consult with a qualified medical practitioner to ensure suitability and safety before engaging in any program outlined herein.

Sources

1. **Oxalate content database based on the latest trustworthy studies**
   ✞ **Link:** https://oxalatecontent.com/
2. Bsc, S.N., NutR, N.G.S.P.N.R., 1999. Oxalate content of foods and its effect on humans. Asia Pacific Journal of Clinical Nutrition 8, 64–74. https://doi.org/10.1046/j.1440-6047.1999.00038.x
3. **Uci Kidneystone Center**
   ✞ **Link:** https://ucikidneystonecenter.com/wpcontent/uploads/2020/06/Oxalate-Content-of-Foods.pdf
4. **Urology Group Virginia**
   ✞ **Link:** https://www.urologygroupvirginia.com/content/kidneystone-center/7-oxalate-and-kidney-stones/oxalate-food-listsummer-2020_3-7-1.pdf
5. **Oxalosis Hyperoxaluria Foundation**
   ✞ **Link:** ohf.org

Contents

INTRODUCTION

If you have been diligently incorporating kale, beets, soy, chia seeds, or green tea into your diet, or know someone who prides themselves on consuming "wholesome" foods like raspberries and buckwheat without experiencing improved health, this book is for you. If you're grappling with persistent symptoms such as gut issues, joint pain, inflammation, kidney stones, rashes, and more, that puzzle your doctors, this book might offer the relief you're seeking.

I am a certified nutritionist and a strong advocate for health and wellness. My journey with oxalates began not through personal suffering, but by witnessing my mother's struggles. Despite consuming what many would consider a perfectly healthy diet, she experienced chronic pain, fatigue, migraines, and other issues. Her journey to wellness, which included identifying and eliminating high-oxalate foods, opened my eyes to the hidden dangers of these so-called health foods.

Many of today's beloved "health foods" can have significant health implications due to oxalates, which are naturally occurring chemical compounds found in many plants. Despite two centuries of scientific evidence, the harmful effects of oxalates remain controversial. It's time to challenge these long-held beliefs and recognize the potential dangers of current food trends.

This book, "**Low Oxalate Food List**," aims to present the science behind the surprising healing responses and gradual recovery that a wellmanaged low-oxalate diet can bring by making informed choices on the foods to eat.

Before the creation of this book, I've delved deep into research and distilled the key findings for you. This book is divided into two parts. **Here's what you'll discover in Part 1 (The Basics) of this book:**

- ✝ What Oxalates Are and Where They Come From, In Our Foods, And in Our Bodies.
- ✝ Misconceptions About Oxalates.
- ✝ How Oxalates Cause Health Problems
- ✝ The Wide Range of Symptoms and Diseases Associated with Oxalate Overload.
- ✝ The Connection Between Oxalates and Calcium
- ✝ The Low Oxalate Diet
- ✝ How to Use This Book

In Part 2, you'll find a carefully curated list of **over 800 food ingredients categorized by their oxalate content**. This section includes individual ingredients and pre-made products, making it easy for you to make informed choices. Each item is clearly listed with its oxalate content, providing a practical guide to help you manage and reduce your oxalate intake effectively.

Part 1
The
Basics

Understanding Oxalates

What Are Oxalates and Where Do They Come From?

Let's begin by diving right into understanding oxalates. You might have heard the term tossed around, but what exactly are oxalates? Oxalates are naturally occurring chemical compounds found in many plants. They serve as a defense mechanism for plants, protecting them from being eaten by pests. But that's not all! Our bodies also produce oxalates as a waste product. Now, these little guys can bind with minerals like calcium, iron, and magnesium to form crystals, and if they accumulate in high amounts, they can lead to health issues like kidney stones. Ouch! So, while oxalates are helpful for plants, they can be problematic for us.

Oxalates in Our Foods

Many foods that contain oxalates are often considered healthy. Leafy greens like beet greens, spinach, and Swiss chard are high in oxalates despite their nutritional benefits. Vegetables such as beets, sweet potatoes, and okra are also staples in many diets and have high oxalate content. Fruits like raspberries, figs, and kiwis are essential for a balanced diet but contain significant levels of oxalates. Nuts and seeds, including almonds, cashews, and chia seeds, are rich in oxalates, making moderation crucial. Popular health foods like dark chocolate, black tea, and quinoa contribute to oxalate intake, emphasizing the need for awareness and balance in our food choices. Oxalates form water-soluble compounds with sodium, potassium, and ammonium ions, but they also bind with calcium, iron, and magnesium, making these minerals unavailable to our bodies. Interestingly, zinc seems to be less affected. Oxalate levels can vary within species; for instance, spinach can have between 400 to 900 mg of oxalic acid per 100 grams. Additionally, oxalic acid tends to accumulate in plants, especially in dry conditions.

Oxalates in Our Bodies

When we consume foods high in oxalates, they bind with minerals such as calcium to form crystals, which can accumulate in various parts of the body and lead to health issues. The most well-known problem is kidney stones, where oxalate crystals form stones in the kidneys, causing severe pain and urinary problems. Oxalates can also accumulate in the joints, causing pain and inflammation similar to arthritis. In the digestive system, oxalates can cause irritation and contribute to issues like irritable bowel syndrome (IBS). Additionally, oxalate crystals can deposit in other tissues, potentially leading to skin rashes, fatigue, and muscle pain. Our bodies also naturally produce a small amount of oxalates as a byproduct of metabolism. While this doesn't cause any significant health problems, the consumption of additional oxalic acid can lead to stone formation in the urinary tract.

What Causes Oxalate Build Up

Oxalate build-up can occur due to a variety of reasons:

Genetic Factors: there is a rare genetic disorder called primary hyperoxaluria. It's like a sneaky saboteur that messes with your liver's ability to produce enough of the right enzymes to keep oxalate production in check.

Sometimes, the enzymes are there, but they're just not doing their job properly.

Gastrointestinal Conditions: Pathological conditions like Crohn's disease and inflammatory bowel disease can lead to a situation called enteric hyperoxaluria. This is when your body starts absorbing more oxalate than it should, leading to too much oxalate in your urine. And guess what? Even conditions that mess with the small intestine's ability to absorb nutrients properly can cause hyperoxaluria.

Dietary Factors: Here's where your diet comes into play. When you consume foods high in oxalate, like spinach, beets, soy, almonds, and potatoes, it can lead to something called dietary hyperoxaluria. It may surprise you to learn that eating a lot of vitamin C might raise the body's oxalate levels. Yes! Vitamin C has a way of converting into oxalate. In fact, when you consume more than 1,000 milligrams of vitamin C per day, it's been shown to ramp up those oxalate levels.

That's not all, though. An increase in oxalate levels in the body can also result from taking antibiotics or having a medical history of digestive disorders. This is the reason why: Our gut's beneficial bacteria operate as oxalate's natural antagonist. They help to kick oxalate out of the body. But when these good bacteria are in short supply, say due to antibiotics or digestive issues, more oxalate can stick around and be absorbed in the body.

Misconceptions About Oxalates

Now we have completed the section on understanding oxalates and where they come from, don't let that scary name fool you. While it's true that they can mess with how our bodies absorb certain nutrients, they're not all bad.

Here's where things get a bit tricky. There are a bunch of misconceptions floating around about oxalates that can cause some unnecessary worry. Let's clear those up:

"Oxalates are the enemy!"

It's a frequent misconception that all oxalates are bad, however this isn't quite accurate. Although some people may develop kidney stones as a result of excessive oxalates, oxalates can actually have both beneficial and detrimental impacts on our health. For instance, oxalates can aid because they bind to excess calcium and stop it from being absorbed. This is especially advantageous for those who have hypercalcemia or certain metabolic diseases.

"Stay away from high-oxalate foods!"

Hold on a second. Many foods that are high in oxalates are also packed with fiber, magnesium, potassium, phytate as well as other highly beneficial nutrients. So, it's all about balance and moderation in the consumption of these foods.

"Oxalates are the Sole Cause of Kidney Stones"

Nope, there's more to the story. While oxalates can contribute to kidney stones, they're not the only factor that contributes to this disease.

"Cooking gets rid of all oxalates"

If only it were that simple that boiling our foods can eliminate oxalates in them, but this is another misconception we need to deal with. Cooking can reduce oxalates, but it doesn't completely get rid of them.

"Avoid calcium to prevent kidney stones"

This one's a bit counterintuitive. Many people think avoiding calcium would help prevent kidney stones since they're made of calcium, but the truth is, if your calcium intake is too low, you're actually at risk of absorbing more oxalate.

How Oxalates Cause Health Problems

Oxalates crystallize when they react with body minerals, especially calcium and iron. If these crystals accumulate excessively, they can cause various health problems.

Symptoms of Oxalate Overload

The symptoms of having too many oxalates in the body can vary widely, depending on the specific health issue they cause. The following are typical indicators to be aware of:

Pain in the back or abdomen: This may indicate kidney stones, which are frequently associated with elevated oxalate levels.

Blood in the urine: Since kidney stones sometimes bleed when they pass, this is another sign of kidney stones.

Urinating frequently: This may be a sign of urinary tract discomfort brought on by oxalate crystals.

Vomiting and nausea: These signs of oxalate poisoning may manifest if oxalate levels are abnormally elevated.

Loss of appetite: This can happen due to the general discomfort and pain caused by high oxalate levels.

Weakness and fatigue: These may indicate a mineral deficiency, since oxalates bind to minerals and interfere with their effective absorption.

Diseases Associated with Oxalate Overload

Kidney Stones

Kidney stones are the most prevalent health issue brought on by elevated oxalate levels. The most prevalent kind of kidney stone is called a calcium oxalate stone, which is created when oxalates in the urine combine with calcium. These stones can be quite painful and may need to be surgically removed.

Mineral Deficiencies

Additionally, oxalates have the ability to bind to other minerals in the body, including magnesium and iron, which might hinder the normal absorption of these nutrients. This may result in mineral shortages, which may give rise to a number of health issues, such as bone loss and anemia.

Oxalate Poisoning

Rarely, oxalate poisoning may result from ingesting abnormally high levels of oxalates. Severe symptoms such as burning in the mouth and throat, breathing difficulties, and in extreme situations, convulsions or unconsciousness, may result from this.

Additional Health Issues

Elevated levels of oxalate have been linked to several health concerns, such as oxidative damage, inflammation, and digestive disorders. Although additional study is required in these areas, some evidence indicates that oxalates may potentially contribute to the development of some chronic disorders, such as vulvodynia and fibromyalgia.

Oxalates and Calcium: A Complex Relationship

The body's bioavailability of several minerals, especially calcium, is greatly impacted by oxalic acid and its salts. As such, oxalic acid has a high tendency to bind with calcium ions (Ca^{2+}). Formed during this reaction is calcium oxalate, which readily dissolves under acidic conditions but is insoluble under a neutral or alkali pH. The formation of calcium oxalate hampers the absorption of calcium by the body. Therefore, overindulging in this type of food can lead to a deficiency of calcium. This means that even if one's diet contains large quantities of calcium, oxalates can substantially reduce its absorption from meals. Spinach, for instance, is an example of a food that has a high content of calcium, but due to its high levels of oxalate, the available amount of calcium absorbed into the body is practically negligible. This resultant compound would be excreted via feces.

WAYS TO REDUCE THE EFFECTS OF OXALATES

It's advisable to eat foods rich in oxalates in moderation and together with foods rich in calcium so as to reduce their impacts on calcium absorption. Boiling food can help lower its level of oxalates, among other cooking methods. This food list in this guidebook includes both lowoxalate-content foods and foods with high calcium content. This is needed to help balance out the formation of calcium oxalates and also increase the body's calcium availability.

The Low Oxalate Diet

The goal of the low-oxalate diet is to reduce the intake of oxalates, which are naturally occurring substances that, if overindulged, can have several negative effects. People who follow this diet are less likely to experience health problems like kidney stones and joint discomfort, which are brought on by excessive oxalates in the diet.

First and foremost, it's critical to understand which foods are high in oxalates. These consist of quinoa, dark chocolate, black tea, and beet greens; almonds, cashews, and chia seeds; beets, sweet potatoes, and okra; raspberries, figs, and kiwi fruits. It is preferable to manage highoxalate foods while, whenever feasible, substituting them with lowoxalate ones rather than completely removing them from your diet. For instance, swap out spinach for bok choy or kale; substitute almonds or cashews for pumpkin or sunflower seeds; and substitute carrots or cucumbers for beets or sweet potatoes.

Increasing the amount of calcium-rich foods you eat at meals is another strategy to help manage the amount of oxalates in your system. In the digestive system, calcium interacts with oxalates to decrease the rate of absorption. Purchase dairy goods like yogurt and milk cheese; lowoxalate veggies like kale; and fortified foods like calcium-rich orange juice. Always stay hydrated. One can avoid kidney stones by preventing the development of urine that contains too much oxalic acid by consuming adequate water. Have eight to ten cups a day.

It's important to keep a balanced diet. To maintain general health while controlling oxalate intake, make sure your diet consists of a range of lowoxalate fruits, vegetables, proteins, and grains.

You will be starting your low-oxalate diet journey with the food list found in part two of this book. You can effectively control and lower potential health concerns linked with high oxalate consumption by adhering to the principles of the low oxalate diet. This diet encourages a well-balanced way of eating, so you can prioritize your health and enjoy a wide range of foods.

How to Use This Book

Welcome to the new and improved edition of the *Low Oxalate Food List*! This guide was created to help you take the guesswork out of managing oxalate intake. Whether you're navigating chronic health symptoms, managing kidney stone risk, or simply aiming to understand your body better, this book is your practical and accurate companion.

What's Different in This Edition

We've listened to reader feedback and made significant upgrades:

- **Every food is now listed with accurate oxalate values per 100g and per serving**

- **Serving sizes are clearly specified in grams and common household measurements**

- **Calculated oxalate content per serving is included for easy tracking**

- **Each food is labeled as Low, Moderate, High, or Very High oxalate based on standard scientific ranges**

These improvements make it easier for you to make informed decisions, compare food options, and build a balanced low-oxalate diet with confidence.

Oxalate Rating System

Each food entry in the list has been categorized using a standardized oxalate classification system based on **oxalate content per serving**:

Oxalate Level	Oxalate per Serving
Very High Oxalate	300 mg or more per serving
High Oxalate	100–299 mg per serving
Moderate Oxalate	25–99 mg per serving
Low Oxalate	Less than 25 mg per serving

You'll see this classification clearly written beneath each food item in the food list.

Understanding Variations in Oxalate Data

Oxalate content can vary slightly depending on food variety, growing conditions, and processing methods. Additionally, various international sources use slightly different classification ranges. For example, some consider foods under **5 mg** per serving as low oxalate, while others go up to **10 mg** or **15 mg**.

To provide consistency and clarity, we've adopted the broader, research-backed range above and verified values using the **Oxalosis and Hyperoxaluria Foundation (OHF) updated list**, among other reputable resources. This ensures you get a reliable, evidence-based reference that's easy to follow.

How to Navigate the Food List (Part 2)

The second half of this book features an **alphabetically organized food list** that includes:

- **Food Name**

- **Oxalate per 100 grams**

- **Serving Size** (in household terms and grams)

- **Calculated Oxalate per Serving**

- **Oxalate Category Label (Low, Moderate, High, Very High)**

Use this section to:

☑ **Plan meals** by choosing mostly low to moderate oxalate foods

☑ **Swap high-oxalate ingredients** with better alternatives

☑ **Track your daily intake** based on the oxalate-per-serving data provided

☑ **Understand packaged foods and ingredients** to help manage oxalate load even when eating out or on the go

Recommended Daily Oxalate Intake

Your ideal oxalate intake depends on your personal health situation. Here are general guidelines:

- **High Risk (e.g., history of kidney stones, hyperoxaluria):**
  Under 50 mg of oxalates per day

- **Moderate Risk:**
  50–100 mg per day

- **Low Risk/General Health:**
  Up to 150 mg per day, ideally spread out and balanced

Consult your healthcare provider or a registered dietitian to determine the best target range for you.

Final Tips

- **Hydration is essential** – aim for 8–10 cups of water daily to help flush oxalates through the urine.

- **Pair oxalate-rich foods with calcium-rich foods** during meals to limit oxalate absorption.

- **Boiling** certain vegetables can significantly reduce their oxalate content.

- **Balance is key** – focus on variety and nutrient density while managing oxalate load.

This book is meant to be a practical, research-based tool that helps you understand and manage oxalates in everyday life. Keep it close—whether you're meal planning, grocery shopping, or simply curious—and feel confident knowing you're making informed decisions for your health.

Note

This food list provides an extensive overview of a wide variety of foods and their corresponding oxalate content. While it aims to be thorough, it may not include every possible food item. Additionally, some items may be unavailable in certain regions or may be known by different names depending on local terminology. Use this guide as a dependable tool for managing your low-oxalate diet, but keep in mind regional differences and availability when making dietary choices.

Part 2

Food List

Adobo or Mexican Adobo

Avg Oxalate per 100 g	Serving Size	Serving (g)	Calculated Oxalate per Serving
41 mg	2 tsp	8 g	3 mg

Remark: Low oxalate food (Less than 25 mg per serving).

Agave Nectar

Avg Oxalate per 100 g	Serving Size	Serving (g)	Calculated Oxalate per Serving
1 mg	1 tbsp	21 g	0 mg

Remark: Low oxalate food (Less than 25 mg per serving).

Alfalfa Sprouts

Avg Oxalate per 100 g	Serving Size	Serving (g)	Calculated Oxalate per Serving
13 mg	½ cup	17 g	2 mg

Remark: Low oxalate food (Less than 25 mg per serving).

Algae and algae derivatives

Avg Oxalate per 100 g	Serving Size	Serving (g)	Calculated Oxalate per Serving
140 mg	2 tbsp	10 g	14 mg

Remark: Low oxalate food (Less than 25 mg per serving).

Algae (dried)

Avg Oxalate per 100 g	Serving Size	Serving (g)	Calculated Oxalate per Serving
109 mg	1 oz	28 g	30 mg

Remark: Moderate oxalate food (25–99 mg per serving)

All-Purpose Flour

Avg Oxalate per 100 g	Serving Size	Serving (g)	Calculated Oxalate per Serving
2 mg	1 cup unsifted	125 g	3 mg

Remark: Low oxalate food (Less than 25 mg per serving).

Almond Extract

Avg Oxalate per 100 g	Serving Size	Serving (g)	Calculated Oxalate per Serving
6 mg	1 tsp	5 g	0 mg

Remark: **Low oxalate food** (Less than 25 mg per serving).

Almond Milk, Commercial (Multi-Brands)

Avg Oxalate per 100 g	Serving Size	Serving (g)	Calculated Oxalate per Serving
10 mg	1 cup	242 g	24 mg

Remark: **Low oxalate food** (Less than 25 mg per serving).
A Calcium-fortified version is always recommended.

Almond Milk, Homemade

(160 g Almonds = 2 cups milk)

Avg Oxalate per 100 g	Serving Size	Serving (g)	Calculated Oxalate per Serving
68 mg	1 cup	242 g	165 mg

Remark: **High oxalate food** (100–299 mg per serving).

Almond Flour

Avg Oxalate per 100 g	Serving Size	Serving (g)	Calculated Oxalate per Serving
519 mg	1/4 cup	38 g	197 mg

Remark: **High oxalate food** (100–299 mg per serving).

Almond Yogurt

All flavors, Multi-Brand

Avg Oxalate per 100 g	Serving Size	Serving (g)	Calculated Oxalate per Serving
39 mg	6 oz	170 g	66 mg

Remark: **Moderate oxalate food** (25–99 mg per serving).

Almonds

Raw or dry roasted

Avg Oxalate per 100 g	Serving Size	Serving (g)	Calculated Oxalate per Serving
369 mg	¼ cup	29 g	107 mg

Remark: **High oxalate food** (100–299 mg per serving).

Amaranth, uncooked

Avg Oxalate per 100 g	Serving Size	Serving (g)	Calculated Oxalate per Serving
151 mg	¼ cup	48.5 g	73 mg

Remark: **Moderate oxalate food** (25–99 mg per serving).

Amaranth Flour

Avg Oxalate per 100 g	Serving Size	Serving (g)	Calculated Oxalate per Serving
283 mg	¼ cup	26 g	74 mg

Remark: **Moderate oxalate food** (25–99 mg per serving).

Anchovy

Avg Oxalate per 100 g	Serving Size	Serving (g)	Calculated Oxalate per Serving
0 mg	2 oz (5 fillets)	56 g	0 mg

Remark: **Low oxalate food** (Less than 25 mg per serving).

Anise

Avg Oxalate per 100 g	Serving Size	Serving (g)	Calculated Oxalate per Serving
951 mg	1 tsp	2.1 g	20 mg

Remark: Low oxalate food (Less than 25 mg per serving).

Apple

Avg Oxalate per 100 g	Serving Size	Serving (g)	Calculated Oxalate per Serving
2 mg	1 medium	138 g	2 mg

Remark: Low oxalate food (Less than 25 mg per serving).

Apple Juice

Avg Oxalate per 100 g	Serving Size	Serving (g)	Calculated Oxalate per Serving
1 mg	1 cup	240 g	1 mg

Remark: Low oxalate food (Less than 25 mg per serving).

Apricot (Dried or Fresh)

Avg Oxalate per 100 g	Serving Size	Serving (g)	Calculated Oxalate per Serving
87 mg	4 x ½ apricots	14 g	12 mg

Remark: **Low oxalate food** (Less than 25 mg per serving).

Apricot Juice

Avg Oxalate per 100 g	Serving Size	Serving (g)	Calculated Oxalate per Serving
2 mg	1 cup	250 g	5 mg

Remark: **Low oxalate food** (Less than 25 mg per serving).

Artichoke (cooked)

Avg Oxalate per 100 g	Serving Size	Serving (g)	Calculated Oxalate per Serving
13 mg	½ cup	84 g	11 mg

Remark: **Low oxalate food** (Less than 25 mg per serving).

Asparagus

Avg Oxalate per 100 g	Serving Size	Serving (g)	Calculated Oxalate per Serving
6 mg	½ cup	90 g	5 mg

Remark: Low oxalate food (Less than 25 mg per serving).

Aspartame (artificial sweetener)

Avg Oxalate per 100 g	Serving Size	Serving (g)	Calculated Oxalate per Serving
4 mg	1 tsp	5 g	0 mg

Remark: Low oxalate food (Less than 25 mg per serving).

Avocado

Avg Oxalate per 100 g	Serving Size	Serving (g)	Calculated Oxalate per Serving
10 mg	½ cup sliced	73 g	7 mg

Remark: Low oxalate food (Less than 25 mg per serving).

Avocado Oil

Avg Oxalate per 100 g	Serving Size	Serving (g)	Calculated Oxalate per Serving
10 mg	1 tbsp	14 g	1 mg

Remark: Low oxalate food (Less than 25 mg per serving).

Aztec Broccoli or Huazontle

Avg Oxalate per 100 g	Serving Size	Serving (g)	Calculated Oxalate per Serving
438 mg	½ cup	60 g	263 mg

Remark: High oxalate food (100–299 mg per serving).

Bacon

Avg Oxalate per 100 g	Serving Size	Serving (g)	Calculated Oxalate per Serving
0 mg	1 slice (1.2 oz)	16 g	0 mg

Remark: Low oxalate food (Less than 25 mg per serving).

Bagel

Avg Oxalate per 100 g	Serving Size	Serving (g)	Calculated Oxalate per Serving
23 mg	1 bagel	95 g	22 mg

Remark: **Low oxalate food** (Less than 25 mg per serving).

Baked Beans

Avg Oxalate per 100 g	Serving Size	Serving (g)	Calculated Oxalate per Serving
13 mg	½ cup	133 g	17 mg

Remark: **Low oxalate food** (Less than 25 mg per serving).

Baking Flour (Gluten Free)

Avg Oxalate per 100 g	Serving Size	Serving (g)	Calculated Oxalate per Serving
19 mg	¼ cup	37 g	7 mg

Remark: **Low oxalate food** (Less than 25 mg per serving).

Bamboo Shoots

Avg Oxalate per 100 g	Serving Size	Serving (g)	Calculated Oxalate per Serving
23 mg	1 cup	151 g	35 mg

Remark: **Moderate oxalate food** (25–99 mg per serving).

Banana Chips

Avg Oxalate per 100 g	Serving Size	Serving (g)	Calculated Oxalate per Serving
203 mg	13 pieces	30 g	61 mg

Remark: **Moderate oxalate food** (25–99 mg per serving).

Bananas

Avg Oxalate per 100 g	Serving Size	Serving (g)	Calculated Oxalate per Serving
5 mg	1 medium	118 g	6 mg

Remark: **Low oxalate food** (Less than 25 mg per serving).

Barbecue Chicken

Avg Oxalate per 100 g	Serving Size	Serving (g)	Calculated Oxalate per Serving
0 mg	1 thigh	95 g	0 mg

Remark: Low oxalate food (Less than 25 mg per serving).

Barley Flour

Avg Oxalate per 100 g	Serving Size	Serving (g)	Calculated Oxalate per Serving
41 mg	¼ cup	35 g	14 mg

Remark: Low oxalate food (Less than 25 mg per serving).

Barley Malt Flour

Avg Oxalate per 100 g	Serving Size	Serving (g)	Calculated Oxalate per Serving
0 mg	½ cup	70 g	0 mg

Remark: Low oxalate food (Less than 25 mg per serving).

Barley Malt Syrup

Avg Oxalate per 100 g	Serving Size	Serving (g)	Calculated Oxalate per Serving
19 mg	1 tbsp	21 g	4 mg

Remark: **Low oxalate food** (Less than 25 mg per serving).

Basil

Avg Oxalate per 100 g	Serving Size	Serving (g)	Calculated Oxalate per Serving
133 mg	1 tsp	2.1 g	3 mg

Remark: **Low oxalate food** (Less than 25 mg per serving).

Basil Wraps

Avg Oxalate per 100 g	Serving Size	Serving (g)	Calculated Oxalate per Serving
25 mg	1 cup	240 g	60 mg

Remark: **Moderate oxalate food** (25–99 mg per serving).

Bay Leaf

Avg Oxalate per 100 g	Serving Size	Serving (g)	Calculated Oxalate per Serving
2744 mg	1 tbsp	1.8 g	49 mg

Remark: **Moderate oxalate food** (25–99 mg per serving).

Bean Soup

Avg Oxalate per 100 g	Serving Size	Serving (g)	Calculated Oxalate per Serving
25 mg	1 cup	164 g	40 mg

Remark: **Moderate oxalate food** (25–99 mg per serving).

Beef Tenderloin

Avg Oxalate per 100 g	Serving Size	Serving (g)	Calculated Oxalate per Serving
0 mg	3 oz	85 g	0 mg

Remark: **Low oxalate food** (Less than 25 mg per serving).

Beef (Roasted)

Avg Oxalate per 100 g	Serving Size	Serving (g)	Calculated Oxalate per Serving
0 mg	1 slice	13.8 g	0 mg

Remark: **Low oxalate food** (Less than 25 mg per serving).

Beef Stroganoff

Avg Oxalate per 100 g	Serving Size	Serving (g)	Calculated Oxalate per Serving
0 mg	1 cup	240 g	0 mg

Remark: **Low oxalate food** (Less than 25 mg per serving).

Beer

Avg Oxalate per 100 g	Serving Size	Serving (g)	Calculated Oxalate per Serving
1 mg	12 oz	356 g	2 mg

Remark: **Low oxalate food** (Less than 25 mg per serving).

Beetroot Juice

Avg Oxalate per 100 g	Serving Size	Serving (g)	Calculated Oxalate per Serving
66 mg	1 cup	250 g	164 mg

Remark: High oxalate food (100–299 mg per serving).

Beets

Avg Oxalate per 100 g	Serving Size	Serving (g)	Calculated Oxalate per Serving
57 mg	½ cup	85 g	48 mg

Remark: Moderate oxalate food (25–99 mg per serving).

Beet Powder

Avg Oxalate per 100 g	Serving Size	Serving (g)	Calculated Oxalate per Serving
997 mg	1 tbsp	10 g	100 mg

Remark: High oxalate food (100–299 mg per serving)

Bell Peppers

Avg Oxalate per 100 g	Serving Size	Serving (g)	Calculated Oxalate per Serving
10 mg	1 medium size	119 g	12 mg

Remark: Low oxalate food (Less than 25 mg per serving).

Biscuit (Breakfast Biscuit, Any Brand)

Avg Oxalate per 100 g	Serving Size	Serving (g)	Calculated Oxalate per Serving
12 mg	1 biscuit	85 g	10 mg

Remark: Low oxalate food (Less than 25 mg per serving).

Bitter Gourd or Bitter Melon

Avg Oxalate per 100 g	Serving Size	Serving (g)	Calculated Oxalate per Serving
86 mg	1 cup	93 g	80 mg

Remark: Moderate oxalate food (25–99 mg per serving).

Bitter Gourd or Bitter Melon Juice

Avg Oxalate per 100 g	Serving Size	Serving (g)	Calculated Oxalate per Serving
27 mg	1 cup	250 g	68 mg

Remark: **Moderate oxalate food** (25–99 mg per serving).

Black Bean and Kale

Avg Oxalate per 100 g	Serving Size	Serving (g)	Calculated Oxalate per Serving
12 mg	1 cup	246 g	29 mg

Remark: **Moderate oxalate food** (25–99 mg per serving).

Black Currant Juice

Avg Oxalate per 100 g	Serving Size	Serving (g)	Calculated Oxalate per Serving
1 mg	1 cup	250 g	3 mg

Remark: **Low oxalate food** (Less than 25 mg per serving).

Black Gram

Avg Oxalate per 100 g	Serving Size	Serving (g)	Calculated Oxalate per Serving
422 mg	1 cup	180 g	760 mg

Remark: **Very high oxalate food** (300 mg or higher per serving).

Black Pepper

Avg Oxalate per 100 g	Serving Size	Serving (g)	Calculated Oxalate per Serving
623 mg	1 tsp	2.3 g	14 mg

Remark: **Low oxalate food** (Less than 25 mg per serving).

Black Tea

Avg Oxalate per 100 g	Serving Size	Serving (g)	Calculated Oxalate per Serving
4.92 mg	6 fl oz	178 g	7 mg

Remark: **Low oxalate food** (Less than 25 mg per serving).

Blackberries

Avg Oxalate per 100 g	Serving Size	Serving (g)	Calculated Oxalate per Serving
31 mg	1 cup	144 g	45 mg

Remark: **Moderate oxalate food** (25–99 mg per serving).

Black-Eyed Peas

Avg Oxalate per 100 g	Serving Size	Serving (g)	Calculated Oxalate per Serving
3 mg	½ cup	86 g	3 mg

Remark: **Low oxalate food** (Less than 25 mg per serving).

Blood Sausage

Avg Oxalate per 100 g	Serving Size	Serving (g)	Calculated Oxalate per Serving
0 mg	4 slices	100 g	0 mg

Remark: **Low oxalate food** (Less than 25 mg per serving).

Blue Cheese

Avg Oxalate per 100 g	Serving Size	Serving (g)	Calculated Oxalate per Serving
0 mg	1 oz	28.35 g	0 mg

Remark: **Low oxalate food** (Less than 25 mg per serving).

Blueberries

Avg Oxalate per 100 g	Serving Size	Serving (g)	Calculated Oxalate per Serving
14 mg	1 cup	200 g	27 mg

Remark: **Moderate oxalate food** (25–99 mg per serving).

Bob's Red Mill Hemp

Avg Oxalate per 100 g	Serving Size	Serving (g)	Calculated Oxalate per Serving
104 mg	1/4 cup	31 g	32 mg

Remark: **Moderate oxalate food** (25–99 mg per serving)

Bok Choy

Avg Oxalate per 100 g	Serving Size	Serving (g)	Calculated Oxalate per Serving
2 mg	1 cup	120 g	2 mg

Remark: **Low oxalate food** (Less than 25 mg per serving).

Bologna Sausage

Avg Oxalate per 100 g	Serving Size	Serving (g)	Calculated Oxalate per Serving
1.4 mg	1 slice	28 g	0 mg

Remark: **Low oxalate food** (Less than 25 mg per serving).

Bran Flakes (Cereal)

Avg Oxalate per 100 g	Serving Size	Serving (g)	Calculated Oxalate per Serving
141 mg	1 cup	35.91 g	51 mg

Remark: **Moderate oxalate food** (25–99 mg per serving).

Bran, Wheat

Avg Oxalate per 100 g	Serving Size	Serving (g)	Calculated Oxalate per Serving
207 mg	¼ cup	14.5 g	30 mg

Remark: Moderate oxalate food (25–99 mg per serving).

Brandy

Avg Oxalate per 100 g	Serving Size	Serving (g)	Calculated Oxalate per Serving
1 mg	1.5 oz	28.4 g	0 mg

Remark: Low oxalate food (Less than 25 mg per serving).

Brazil Nut

Avg Oxalate per 100 g	Serving Size	Serving (g)	Calculated Oxalate per Serving
181 mg	¼ cup	29 g	52 mg

Remark: Moderate oxalate food (25–99 mg per serving).

Bread

Avg Oxalate per 100 g	Serving Size	Serving (g)	Calculated Oxalate per Serving
23 mg	1 bagel	95 g	22 mg

Remark: **Low oxalate food** (Less than 25 mg per serving).

Bread (from Organic Seeds and Grains)

Avg Oxalate per 100 g	Serving Size	Serving (g)	Calculated Oxalate per Serving
112 mg	1 slice	38 g	42 mg

Remark: **Moderate oxalate food** (25–99 mg per serving).

Brie

Avg Oxalate per 100 g	Serving Size	Serving (g)	Calculated Oxalate per Serving
0 mg	1 oz	28.35 g	0 mg

Remark: **Low oxalate food** (Less than 25 mg per serving).

Broccoli (Raw)

Avg Oxalate per 100 g	Serving Size	Serving (g)	Calculated Oxalate per Serving
12 mg	1 cup	80 g	9 mg

Remark: Low oxalate food (Less than 25 mg per serving).

Broccoli (Cooked)

Avg Oxalate per 100 g	Serving Size	Serving (g)	Calculated Oxalate per Serving
7 mg	½ cup	60 g	4 mg

Remark: Low oxalate food (Less than 25 mg per serving).

Brown Rice

Avg Oxalate per 100 g	Serving Size	Serving (g)	Calculated Oxalate per Serving
6 mg	½ cup	90 g	5 mg

Remark: Low oxalate food (Less than 25 mg per serving).

Brown Rice Syrup

Avg Oxalate per 100 g	Serving Size	Serving (g)	Calculated Oxalate per Serving
14 mg	2 tbsp	30 g	4 mg

Remark: Low oxalate food (Less than 25 mg per serving).

Brown Sugar

Avg Oxalate per 100 g	Serving Size	Serving (g)	Calculated Oxalate per Serving
11 mg	1 tsp	4.6 g	1 mg

Remark: Low oxalate food (Less than 25 mg per serving).

Brownies

Avg Oxalate per 100 g	Serving Size	Serving (g)	Calculated Oxalate per Serving
85 mg	2 items	27.6 g	23 mg

Remark: Low oxalate food (Less than 25 mg per serving).

Brunost

Avg Oxalate per 100 g	Serving Size	Serving (g)	Calculated Oxalate per Serving
0 mg	1 oz	28.35 g	0 mg

Remark: **Low oxalate food** (Less than 25 mg per serving).

Brussels Sprout

Avg Oxalate per 100 g	Serving Size	Serving (g)	Calculated Oxalate per Serving
15 mg	1 cup	90 g	14 mg

Remark: **Low oxalate food** (Less than 25 mg per serving).

Buckwheat

Avg Oxalate per 100 g	Serving Size	Serving (g)	Calculated Oxalate per Serving
133 mg	1 cup	168 g	223 mg

Remark: **High oxalate food** (100–299 mg per serving).

Buckwheat (Cereal)

Avg Oxalate per 100 g	Serving Size	Serving (g)	Calculated Oxalate per Serving
123 mg	½ cup	85 g	105 mg

Remark: **High oxalate food** (100–299 mg per serving).

Buckwheat Flour

Avg Oxalate per 100 g	Serving Size	Serving (g)	Calculated Oxalate per Serving
280 mg	¼ cup	30 g	84 mg

Remark: **Moderate oxalate food** (25–99 mg per serving).

Bulgur

Avg Oxalate per 100 g	Serving Size	Serving (g)	Calculated Oxalate per Serving
59 mg	1 cup	182 g	107 mg

Remark: **High oxalate food** (100–299 mg per serving).

Butter (Cashew)

Avg Oxalate per 100 g	Serving Size	Serving (g)	Calculated Oxalate per Serving
218 mg	2 tbsp	29 g	63 mg

Remark: **Moderate oxalate food** (25–99 mg per serving).

Butter (Peanut)

Avg Oxalate per 100 g	Serving Size	Serving (g)	Calculated Oxalate per Serving
125 mg	2 tbsp	29 g	36 mg

Remark: **Moderate oxalate food** (25–99 mg per serving).

Buttercrisp Crackers

Avg Oxalate per 100 g	Serving Size	Serving (g)	Calculated Oxalate per Serving
24 mg	5 crackers	16 g	4 mg

Remark: **Low oxalate food** (Less than 25 mg per serving).

Buttermilk

Avg Oxalate per 100 g	Serving Size	Serving (g)	Calculated Oxalate per Serving
0.3 mg	1 cup	245 g	1 mg

Remark: Low oxalate food (Less than 25 mg per serving).

Cabbage

Avg Oxalate per 100 g	Serving Size	Serving (g)	Calculated Oxalate per Serving
5 mg	1 cup	70 g	4 mg

Remark: Low oxalate food (Less than 25 mg per serving).

Candy with Peanuts

Avg Oxalate per 100 g	Serving Size	Serving (g)	Calculated Oxalate per Serving
46 mg	10 pieces	24 g	11 mg

Remark: Low oxalate food (Less than 25 mg per serving).

Cantaloupe

Avg Oxalate per 100 g	Serving Size	Serving (g)	Calculated Oxalate per Serving
0 mg	1 cup	182 g	0 mg

Remark: Low oxalate food (Less than 25 mg per serving).

Capers

Avg Oxalate per 100 g	Serving Size	Serving (g)	Calculated Oxalate per Serving
6 mg	1 tbsp	15 g	1 mg

Remark: Low oxalate food (Less than 25 mg per serving).

Carambola (Starfruit)

Avg Oxalate per 100 g	Serving Size	Serving (g)	Calculated Oxalate per Serving
295 mg	1 medium fruit	91 g	269 mg

Remark: High oxalate food (100–299 mg per serving).

Caraway Seeds

Avg Oxalate per 100 g	Serving Size	Serving (g)	Calculated Oxalate per Serving
863 mg	1 tsp	2.1 g	18 mg

Remark: Low oxalate food (Less than 25 mg per serving).

Cardamom

Avg Oxalate per 100 g	Serving Size	Serving (g)	Calculated Oxalate per Serving
307 mg	1 tsp	2 g	6 mg

Remark: Low oxalate food (Less than 25 mg per serving).

Carrot Juice

Avg Oxalate per 100 g	Serving Size	Serving (g)	Calculated Oxalate per Serving
9 mg	1 cup	250 g	23 mg

Remark: Low oxalate food (Less than 25 mg per serving).

Carrots (Cooked)

Avg Oxalate per 100 g	Serving Size	Serving (g)	Calculated Oxalate per Serving
12 mg	½ cup	78 g	9 mg

Remark: **Low oxalate food** (Less than 25 mg per serving).

Carrots (Raw, Grated)

Avg Oxalate per 100 g	Serving Size	Serving (g)	Calculated Oxalate per Serving
24 mg	1 cup, grated	128 g	30 mg

Remark: **Moderate oxalate food** (25–99 mg per serving).

Cashew (Whole)

Avg Oxalate per 100 g	Serving Size	Serving (g)	Calculated Oxalate per Serving
265 mg	1 oz	28.35 g	75 mg

Remark: **Moderate oxalate food** (25–99 mg per serving).

Cashew Nut Butter

Avg Oxalate per 100 g	Serving Size	Serving (g)	Calculated Oxalate per Serving
218 mg	2 tbsp	29 g	63 mg

Remark: **Moderate oxalate food** (25–99 mg per serving).

Cashew Nut

Avg Oxalate per 100 g	Serving Size	Serving (g)	Calculated Oxalate per Serving
249 mg	¼ cup	29 g	72 mg

Remark: **Moderate oxalate food** (25–99 mg per serving).

Cassava

Avg Oxalate per 100 g	Serving Size	Serving (g)	Calculated Oxalate per Serving
1260 mg	1 cup	206 g	2596 mg

Remark: **Very high oxalate food** (300 mg or higher per serving).

Cassava Flour

Avg Oxalate per 100 g	Serving Size	Serving (g)	Calculated Oxalate per Serving
61 mg	¼ cup	32 g	19 mg

Remark: **Low oxalate food** (Less than 25 mg per serving).

Catfish

Avg Oxalate per 100 g	Serving Size	Serving (g)	Calculated Oxalate per Serving
0.1 mg	3 oz	85 g	0 mg

Remark: **Low oxalate food** (Less than 25 mg per serving).

Cauliflower

Avg Oxalate per 100 g	Serving Size	Serving (g)	Calculated Oxalate per Serving
3 mg	½ cup	60 g	2 mg

Remark: **Low oxalate food** (Less than 25 mg per serving).

Cayenne Pepper

Avg Oxalate per 100 g	Serving Size	Serving (g)	Calculated Oxalate per Serving
20 mg	1 medium	3.5 g	1 mg

Remark: **Low oxalate food** (Less than 25 mg per serving).

Celeriac

Avg Oxalate per 100 g	Serving Size	Serving (g)	Calculated Oxalate per Serving
7 mg	1 cup	156 g	11 mg

Remark: **Low oxalate food** (Less than 25 mg per serving).

Celery (Cooked)

Avg Oxalate per 100 g	Serving Size	Serving (g)	Calculated Oxalate per Serving
25 mg	1 cup	120 g	30 mg

Remark: **Moderate oxalate food** (25–99 mg per serving).

Celery Seeds

Avg Oxalate per 100 g	Serving Size	Serving (g)	Calculated Oxalate per Serving
1274 mg	1 tsp	2.5 g	32 mg

Remark: **Moderate oxalate food** (25–99 mg per serving).

Chayote

Avg Oxalate per 100 g	Serving Size	Serving (g)	Calculated Oxalate per Serving
8 mg	½ cup	80 g	6 mg

Remark: **Low oxalate food** (Less than 25 mg per serving).

Cheddar Cheese

Avg Oxalate per 100 g	Serving Size	Serving (g)	Calculated Oxalate per Serving
0 mg	1 oz	28.35 g	0 mg

Remark: **Low oxalate food** (Less than 25 mg per serving).

Cherries

Avg Oxalate per 100 g	Serving Size	Serving (g)	Calculated Oxalate per Serving
3 mg	1 cup	98 g	2 mg

Remark: **Low oxalate food** (Less than 25 mg per serving).

Cherry Juice

Avg Oxalate per 100 g	Serving Size	Serving (g)	Calculated Oxalate per Serving
1 mg	1 cup	250 g	3 mg

Remark: **Low oxalate food** (Less than 25 mg per serving).

Chestnut

Avg Oxalate per 100 g	Serving Size	Serving (g)	Calculated Oxalate per Serving
28 mg	¼ cup	28.4 g	8 mg

Remark: **Low oxalate food** (Less than 25 mg per serving).

Chia Seed

Avg Oxalate per 100 g	Serving Size	Serving (g)	Calculated Oxalate per Serving
470 mg	1 tbsp	13 g	61 mg

Remark: **Moderate oxalate food** (25–99 mg per serving).

Chicken

Avg Oxalate per 100 g	Serving Size	Serving (g)	Calculated Oxalate per Serving
0.2 mg	3 oz	85 g	0 mg

Remark: **Low oxalate food** (Less than 25 mg per serving).

Chicken Noodle Soup

Avg Oxalate per 100 g	Serving Size	Serving (g)	Calculated Oxalate per Serving
1 mg	1 cup	245 g	2 mg

Remark: **Low oxalate food** (Less than 25 mg per serving).

Chicken Liver

Avg Oxalate per 100 g	Serving Size	Serving (g)	Calculated Oxalate per Serving
0.4 mg	1 liver	44 g	0 mg

Remark: Low oxalate food (Less than 25 mg per serving).

Chicken Salad

Avg Oxalate per 100 g	Serving Size	Serving (g)	Calculated Oxalate per Serving
13 mg	1 entrée	41.3 g	6 mg

Remark: Low oxalate food (Less than 25 mg per serving).

Chickpea Flour

Avg Oxalate per 100 g	Serving Size	Serving (g)	Calculated Oxalate per Serving
10 mg	¼ cup	23 g	2 mg

Remark: Low oxalate food (Less than 25 mg per serving).

Chickpeas

Avg Oxalate per 100 g	Serving Size	Serving (g)	Calculated Oxalate per Serving
10 mg	½ cup	86 g	9 mg

Remark: Low oxalate food (Less than 25 mg per serving).

Chicory

Avg Oxalate per 100 g	Serving Size	Serving (g)	Calculated Oxalate per Serving
210 mg	½ cup	45 g	95 mg

Remark: Moderate oxalate food (25–99 mg per serving).

Chiles

Avg Oxalate per 100 g	Serving Size	Serving (g)	Calculated Oxalate per Serving
51 mg	1 tsp	2 g	1 mg

Remark: Low oxalate food (Less than 25 mg per serving).

Chili Pepper

Avg Oxalate per 100 g	Serving Size	Serving (g)	Calculated Oxalate per Serving
312 mg	1 tsp	2.6 g	8 mg

Remark: **Low oxalate food** (Less than 25 mg per serving).

Chinese Cabbage

Avg Oxalate per 100 g	Serving Size	Serving (g)	Calculated Oxalate per Serving
15 mg	1 cup (shredded)	70 g	11 mg

Remark: **Low oxalate food (Less** than 25 mg per serving).

Chipotle Chili

Avg Oxalate per 100 g	Serving Size	Serving (g)	Calculated Oxalate per Serving
150 mg	1 tsp	2 g	3 mg

Remark: **Low oxalate food** (Less than 25 mg per serving).

Chives

Avg Oxalate per 100 g	Serving Size	Serving (g)	Calculated Oxalate per Serving
5 mg	¼ cup, chopped	12 g	1 mg

Remark: **Low oxalate food** (Less than 25 mg per serving).

Chocolate Chip Cookies

Avg Oxalate per 100 g	Serving Size	Serving (g)	Calculated Oxalate per Serving
37.5 mg	1 cookie	16 g	6.5 mg

Remark: **Low oxalate food** (Less than 25 mg per serving).

Chocolate Milk

Avg Oxalate per 100 g	Serving Size	Serving (g)	Calculated Oxalate per Serving
58 mg	1 cup	250 g	145 mg

Remark: **High oxalate food** (100–299 mg per serving).

Chocolate Syrup

Avg Oxalate per 100 g	Serving Size	Serving (g)	Calculated Oxalate per Serving
2 mg	¼ cup	60 g	1 mg

Remark: Low oxalate food (Less than 25 mg per serving).

Chorizo

Avg Oxalate per 100 g	Serving Size	Serving (g)	Calculated Oxalate per Serving
0 mg	1 oz	28.35 g	0 mg

Remark: Low oxalate food (Less than 25 mg per serving).

Chutney

Avg Oxalate per 100 g	Serving Size	Serving (g)	Calculated Oxalate per Serving
32 mg	1 tbsp	19 g	6 mg

Remark: Low oxalate food (Less than 25 mg per serving).

Cinnamon

Avg Oxalate per 100 g	Serving Size	Serving (g)	Calculated Oxalate per Serving
1072 mg	1 tsp	2.3 g	25 mg

Remark: **Moderate oxalate food** (25–99 mg per serving).

Clam (Cooked)

Avg Oxalate per 100 g	Serving Size	Serving (g)	Calculated Oxalate per Serving
0.1 mg	3 oz	85 g	0 mg

Remark: **Low oxalate food** (Less than 25 mg per serving).

Coca-Cola

Avg Oxalate per 100 g	Serving Size	Serving (g)	Calculated Oxalate per Serving
0 mg	16 fl oz (small)	347 g	0 mg

Remark: **Low oxalate food** (Less than 25 mg per serving).

Cocoa Powder (Not Dutch Process)

Avg Oxalate per 100 g	Serving Size	Serving (g)	Calculated Oxalate per Serving
656 mg	2 tbsp	12 g	79 mg

Remark: **Moderate oxalate food** (25–99 mg per serving).

Cocoa Powder (Dutch Process)

Avg Oxalate per 100 g	Serving Size	Serving (g)	Calculated Oxalate per Serving
170 mg	2 tbsp	12 g	20 mg

Remark: **Low oxalate food** (Less than 25 mg per serving).

Cocoa Solids

Avg Oxalate per 100 g	Serving Size	Serving (g)	Calculated Oxalate per Serving
619 mg	1 cup	86 g	532 mg

Remark: **Very high oxalate food** (300 mg or higher per serving).

Cocoa Bean

Avg Oxalate per 100 g	Serving Size	Serving (g)	Calculated Oxalate per Serving
783 mg	1 cup	86 g	673 mg

Remark: **Very high oxalate food** (300 mg or higher per serving).

Coconut (Shredded)

Avg Oxalate per 100 g	Serving Size	Serving (g)	Calculated Oxalate per Serving
7 mg	1 cup (shredded)	80 g	6 mg

Remark: **Low oxalate food** (Less than 25 mg per serving).

Coconut Flour

Avg Oxalate per 100 g	Serving Size	Serving (g)	Calculated Oxalate per Serving
9 mg	¼ cup	26 g	2 mg

Remark: **Low oxalate food** (Less than 25 mg per serving).

Coconut Milk

Avg Oxalate per 100 g	Serving Size	Serving (g)	Calculated Oxalate per Serving
0 mg	1 cup	242 g	0 mg

Remark: **Low oxalate food** (Less than 25 mg per serving).

Coconut Water

Avg Oxalate per 100 g	Serving Size	Serving (g)	Calculated Oxalate per Serving
7 mg	1 cup	240 g	17 mg

Remark: **Low oxalate food** (Less than 25 mg per serving).

Cod

Avg Oxalate per 100 g	Serving Size	Serving (g)	Calculated Oxalate per Serving
0 mg	1 fillet	185 g	0 mg

Remark: **Low oxalate food** (Less than 25 mg per serving).

Coffee (Black)

Avg Oxalate per 100 g	Serving Size	Serving (g)	Calculated Oxalate per Serving
1 mg	1 cup	236 g	2 mg

Remark: Low oxalate food (Less than 25 mg per serving).

Coffee Mate (Nestlé)

Avg Oxalate per 100 g	Serving Size	Serving (g)	Calculated Oxalate per Serving
4 mg	1 tbsp	15 g	1 mg

Remark: Low oxalate food (Less than 25 mg per serving).

Collard Greens (Raw)

Avg Oxalate per 100 g	Serving Size	Serving (g)	Calculated Oxalate per Serving
17 mg	1 cup	36 g	6 mg

Remark: Low oxalate food (Less than 25 mg per serving).

Collards (Cooked)

Avg Oxalate per 100 g	Serving Size	Serving (g)	Calculated Oxalate per Serving
22 mg	½ cup	95 g	21 mg

Remark: Low oxalate food (Less than 25 mg per serving).

Condensed Milk

Avg Oxalate per 100 g	Serving Size	Serving (g)	Calculated Oxalate per Serving
0 mg	1 cup	306 g	0 mg

Remark: Low oxalate food (Less than 25 mg per serving).

Coriander Seeds

Avg Oxalate per 100 g	Serving Size	Serving (g)	Calculated Oxalate per Serving
1031 mg	1 tsp	1.8 g	19 mg

Remark: Low oxalate food (Less than 25 mg per serving).

Corn (Boiled)

Avg Oxalate per 100 g	Serving Size	Serving (g)	Calculated Oxalate per Serving
3 mg	½ cup	82 g	2 mg

Remark: Low oxalate food (Less than 25 mg per serving).

Corn Flour

Avg Oxalate per 100 g	Serving Size	Serving (g)	Calculated Oxalate per Serving
3 mg	½ cup	60 g	2 mg

Remark: Low oxalate food (Less than 25 mg per serving).

Corn Grits

Avg Oxalate per 100 g	Serving Size	Serving (g)	Calculated Oxalate per Serving
26 mg	½ cup	74.4 g	19 mg

Remark: Low oxalate food (Less than 25 mg per serving).

Cornmeal

Avg Oxalate per 100 g	Serving Size	Serving (g)	Calculated Oxalate per Serving
54 mg	1 cup	157 g	85 mg

Remark: **Moderate oxalate food (**25–99 mg per serving).

Corn Syrup

Avg Oxalate per 100 g	Serving Size	Serving (g)	Calculated Oxalate per Serving
0 mg	1 tbsp	21 g	0 mg

Remark: **Low oxalate food (**Less than 25 mg per serving).

Cornbread

Avg Oxalate per 100 g	Serving Size	Serving (g)	Calculated Oxalate per Serving
9 mg	1 slice	40 g	3 mg

Remark: **Low oxalate food (**Less than 25 mg per serving).

Corned Beef

Avg Oxalate per 100 g	Serving Size	Serving (g)	Calculated Oxalate per Serving
0 mg	3 oz	85 g	0 mg

Remark: Low oxalate food (Less than 25 mg per serving).

Cornstarch

Avg Oxalate per 100 g	Serving Size	Serving (g)	Calculated Oxalate per Serving
3 mg	1 tbsp	8 g	0 mg

Remark: Low oxalate food (Less than 25 mg per serving).

Cotija Cheese

Avg Oxalate per 100 g	Serving Size	Serving (g)	Calculated Oxalate per Serving
0 mg	2 tsp	5 g	0 mg

Remark: Low oxalate food (Less than 25 mg per serving).

Cottage Cheese

Avg Oxalate per 100 g	Serving Size	Serving (g)	Calculated Oxalate per Serving
0 mg	½ cup	113 g	0 mg

Remark: **Low oxalate food** (Less than 25 mg per serving).

Cow Milk

Avg Oxalate per 100 g	Serving Size	Serving (g)	Calculated Oxalate per Serving
1 mg	1 cup	242 g	1 mg

Remark: **Low oxalate food** (Less than 25 mg per serving).

Cracker

Avg Oxalate per 100 g	Serving Size	Serving (g)	Calculated Oxalate per Serving
39 mg	5 crackers	16 g	6 mg

Remark: **Low oxalate food** (Less than 25 mg per serving).

Cranberries

Avg Oxalate per 100 g	Serving Size	Serving (g)	Calculated Oxalate per Serving
4 mg	1 cup	240 g	9 mg

Remark: **Low oxalate food** (Less than 25 mg per serving).

Cranberry Juice

Avg Oxalate per 100 g	Serving Size	Serving (g)	Calculated Oxalate per Serving
1 mg	1 cup	240 g	3 mg

Remark: **Low oxalate food** (Less than 25 mg per serving).

Cream Cheese

Avg Oxalate per 100 g	Serving Size	Serving (g)	Calculated Oxalate per Serving
0.1 mg	1 tbsp	14.5 g	0 mg

Remark: **Low oxalate food** (Less than 25 mg per serving).

Cream of Tartar

Avg Oxalate per 100 g	Serving Size	Serving (g)	Calculated Oxalate per Serving
80 mg	1 tsp	3 g	2 mg

Remark: Low oxalate food (Less than 25 mg per serving).

Cress (Spices)

Avg Oxalate per 100 g	Serving Size	Serving (g)	Calculated Oxalate per Serving
0 mg	1 tsp	1.4 g	0 mg

Remark: Low oxalate food (Less than 25 mg per serving).

Croaker

Avg Oxalate per 100 g	Serving Size	Serving (g)	Calculated Oxalate per Serving
0 mg	1 fillet	87 g	0 mg

Remark: Low oxalate food (Less than 25 mg per serving).

Cucumber

Avg Oxalate per 100 g	Serving Size	Serving (g)	Calculated Oxalate per Serving
4 mg	1 cup, sliced	120 g	5 mg

Remark: **Low oxalate food** (Less than 25 mg per serving).

Cumin

Avg Oxalate per 100 g	Serving Size	Serving (g)	Calculated Oxalate per Serving
1100 mg	1 tsp	2.1 g	23 mg

Remark: **Low oxalate food (**Less than 25 mg per serving).

Currants (Red or Black)

Avg Oxalate per 100 g	Serving Size	Serving (g)	Calculated Oxalate per Serving
19 mg	1 cup	112 g	21 mg

Remark: **Low oxalate food** (Less than 25 mg per serving).

Curry Powder

Avg Oxalate per 100 g	Serving Size	Serving (g)	Calculated Oxalate per Serving
951 mg	1 tsp	2 g	19 mg

Remark: Low oxalate food (Less than 25 mg per serving).

Dandelion Greens

Avg Oxalate per 100 g	Serving Size	Serving (g)	Calculated Oxalate per Serving
22 mg	½ cup, chopped	45 g	10 mg

Remark: Low oxalate food (Less than 25 mg per serving).

Dark Chocolate Candy

Avg Oxalate per 100 g	Serving Size	Serving (g)	Calculated Oxalate per Serving
232 mg	1 oz	28 g	65 mg

Remark: Moderate oxalate food (25–99 mg per serving)

Dark Chocolate Latte

Avg Oxalate per 100 g	Serving Size	Serving (g)	Calculated Oxalate per Serving
20 mg	1 cup	224 g	45 mg

Remark: **Moderate oxalate food** (25–99 mg per serving).

Dates

Avg Oxalate per 100 g	Serving Size	Serving (g)	Calculated Oxalate per Serving
8 mg	¼ cup	45 g	4 mg

Remark: **Low oxalate food** (Less than 25 mg per serving).

Dill (Fresh)

Avg Oxalate per 100 g	Serving Size	Serving (g)	Calculated Oxalate per Serving
145 mg	1 tsp	2.1 g	3 mg

Remark: **Low oxalate food** (Less than 25 mg per serving).

Dried Dill Weed

Avg Oxalate per 100 g	Serving Size	Serving (g)	Calculated Oxalate per Serving
650 mg	1 tsp	1 g	5 mg

Remark: Low oxalate food (Less than 25 mg per serving).

Dried Parsley

Avg Oxalate per 100 g	Serving Size	Serving (g)	Calculated Oxalate per Serving
1127 mg	1 tsp	0.3 g	3 mg

Remark: Low oxalate food (Less than 25 mg per serving).

Duck

Avg Oxalate per 100 g	Serving Size	Serving (g)	Calculated Oxalate per Serving
0 mg	1 cup (chopped)	145 g	0 mg

Remark: Low oxalate food (Less than 25 mg per serving).

Edam (Cheese)

Avg Oxalate per 100 g	Serving Size	Serving (g)	Calculated Oxalate per Serving
0 mg	1 oz	28.35 g	0 mg

Remark: Low oxalate food (Less than 25 mg per serving).

Edamame

Avg Oxalate per 100 g	Serving Size	Serving (g)	Calculated Oxalate per Serving
30 mg	½ cup	75 g	22 mg

Remark: Low oxalate food (Less than 25 mg per serving).

Egg (Whole)

Avg Oxalate per 100 g	Serving Size	Serving (g)	Calculated Oxalate per Serving
0 mg	1 egg equivalent	65 g	0 mg

Remark: Low oxalate food (Less than 25 mg per serving).

Eggnog

Avg Oxalate per 100 g	Serving Size	Serving (g)	Calculated Oxalate per Serving
0 mg	1 fl oz	31.8 g	0 mg

Remark: Low oxalate food (Less than 25 mg per serving).

Eggplant

Avg Oxalate per 100 g	Serving Size	Serving (g)	Calculated Oxalate per Serving
62 mg	½ cup	42 g	26 mg

Remark: Moderate oxalate food (25–99 mg per serving).

Egg Noodles

Avg Oxalate per 100 g	Serving Size	Serving (g)	Calculated Oxalate per Serving
1 mg	1 cup	160 g	2 mg

Remark: Low oxalate food (Less than 25 mg per serving).

Elderberries (Dried)

Avg Oxalate per 100 g	Serving Size	Serving (g)	Calculated Oxalate per Serving
316 mg	2 tbsp	16 g	51 mg

Remark: **Moderate oxalate food** (25–99 mg per serving).

Elderberries (Raw)

Avg Oxalate per 100 g	Serving Size	Serving (g)	Calculated Oxalate per Serving
72 mg	1 cup	145 g	105 mg

Remark: **High oxalate food** (100–299 mg per serving).

Endive

Avg Oxalate per 100 g	Serving Size	Serving (g)	Calculated Oxalate per Serving
5 mg	1 cup, chopped	50 g	3 mg

Remark: **Low oxalate food** (Less than 25 mg per serving).

English Muffin (White)

Avg Oxalate per 100 g	Serving Size	Serving (g)	Calculated Oxalate per Serving
21 mg	1 muffin	60 g	13 mg

Remark: **Low oxalate food** (Less than 25 mg per serving).

English Muffin (Whole Grain)

Avg Oxalate per 100 g	Serving Size	Serving (g)	Calculated Oxalate per Serving
21 mg	1 muffin	60 g	13 mg

Remark: **Low oxalate food** (Less than 25 mg per serving).

Escarole

Avg Oxalate per 100 g	Serving Size	Serving (g)	Calculated Oxalate per Serving
6 mg	1 cup, chopped	40 g	2 mg

Remark: **Low oxalate food** (Less than 25 mg per serving).

Farina Cereal

Avg Oxalate per 100 g	Serving Size	Serving (g)	Calculated Oxalate per Serving
59 mg	1 cup	36.5 g	16 mg

Remark: **Low oxalate food** (Less than 25 mg per serving).

Fat-Free Milk

Avg Oxalate per 100 g	Serving Size	Serving (g)	Calculated Oxalate per Serving
0.3 mg	1 cup	240 g	1 mg

Remark: **Low oxalate food** (Less than 25 mg per serving).

Fava Beans

Avg Oxalate per 100 g	Serving Size	Serving (g)	Calculated Oxalate per Serving
22 mg	½ cup	85 g	18 mg

Remark: **Low oxalate food** (Less than 25 mg per serving).

Fennel (Cooked)

Avg Oxalate per 100 g	Serving Size	Serving (g)	Calculated Oxalate per Serving
5 mg	1 bulb	218 g	12 mg

Remark: **Low oxalate food** (Less than 25 mg per serving).

Fennel Seeds

Avg Oxalate per 100 g	Serving Size	Serving (g)	Calculated Oxalate per Serving
1293 mg	1 tsp	1.8 g	23 mg

Remark: **Low oxalate food** (Less than 25 mg per serving).

Fenugreek

Avg Oxalate per 100 g	Serving Size	Serving (g)	Calculated Oxalate per Serving
1246 mg	1 tbsp	11.2 g	139 mg

Remark: **High oxalate food** (100–299 mg per serving).

Feta

Avg Oxalate per 100 g	Serving Size	Serving (g)	Calculated Oxalate per Serving
0 mg	1 oz	28.35 g	0 mg

Remark: **Low oxalate food** (Less than 25 mg per serving).

Fettuccine Pasta (Organic Spinach Fettuccine)

Avg Oxalate per 100 g	Serving Size	Serving (g)	Calculated Oxalate per Serving
98 mg	1 cup cooked	112 g	109 mg

Remark: **High oxalate food** (100–299 mg per serving).

Fettuccine Pasta (Miracle Noodles)

Avg Oxalate per 100 g	Serving Size	Serving (g)	Calculated Oxalate per Serving
2 mg	3 oz	85 g	2 mg

Remark: **Low oxalate food** (Less than 25 mg per serving).

Fiber One (Cereal)

Avg Oxalate per 100 g	Serving Size	Serving (g)	Calculated Oxalate per Serving
63 mg	1 cup	54.42 g	34 mg

Remark: **Moderate oxalate food** (25–99 mg per serving).

Fig Bars

Avg Oxalate per 100 g	Serving Size	Serving (g)	Calculated Oxalate per Serving
7 mg	1 cookie	50 g	4 mg

Remark: **Low oxalate food** (Less than 25 mg per serving).

Figs (Fresh)

Avg Oxalate per 100 g	Serving Size	Serving (g)	Calculated Oxalate per Serving
21.1 mg	1 medium fig	50 g	11 mg

Remark: **Low oxalate food** (Less than 25 mg per serving)

Figs (Dried)

Avg Oxalate per 100 g	Serving Size	Serving (g)	Calculated Oxalate per Serving
76 mg	1 fig	8.4 g	6 mg

Remark: **Low oxalate food** (Less than 25 mg per serving).

Flax Milk

Avg Oxalate per 100 g	Serving Size	Serving (g)	Calculated Oxalate per Serving
0 mg	1 cup	242 g	0 mg

Remark: **Low oxalate food** (Less than 25 mg per serving).

Flaxseed

Avg Oxalate per 100 g	Serving Size	Serving (g)	Calculated Oxalate per Serving
9 mg	2 tbsp	20 g	2 mg

Remark: **Low oxalate food** (Less than 25 mg per serving).

French Fries (Most Fast-Food Restaurants)

Avg Oxalate per 100 g	Serving Size	Serving (g)	Calculated Oxalate per Serving
30 mg	1 small serving	100 g	30 mg

Remark: **Moderate oxalate food** (25–99 mg per serving).

Fruit Cocktail

Avg Oxalate per 100 g	Serving Size	Serving (g)	Calculated Oxalate per Serving
6 mg	½ cup	95 g	6 mg

Remark: **Low oxalate food** (Less than 25 mg per serving).

Fruit Pectin

Avg Oxalate per 100 g	Serving Size	Serving (g)	Calculated Oxalate per Serving
6 mg	1 tsp	4 g	0 mg

Remark: **Low oxalate food** (Less than 25 mg per serving)

Fruitcake

Avg Oxalate per 100 g	Serving Size	Serving (g)	Calculated Oxalate per Serving
12 mg	1 oz	28.35 g	3 mg

Remark: **Low oxalate food** (Less than 25 mg per serving). Depending on the fruits contained, it can also have a high oxalate value.

Fudge Brownie

Avg Oxalate per 100 g	Serving Size	Serving (g)	Calculated Oxalate per Serving
86 mg	1 brownie (2 in. sq)	24 g	21 mg

Remark: **Low oxalate food** (Less than 25 mg per serving).

Garbanzo Beans

Avg Oxalate per 100 g	Serving Size	Serving (g)	Calculated Oxalate per Serving
10 mg	½ cup	86 g	9 mg

Remark: **Low oxalate food** (Less than 25 mg per serving).

Garden Cress

Avg Oxalate per 100 g	Serving Size	Serving (g)	Calculated Oxalate per Serving
134 mg	1 cup	50 g	67 mg

Remark: Moderate oxalate food (25–99 mg per serving).

Garlic

Avg Oxalate per 100 g	Serving Size	Serving (g)	Calculated Oxalate per Serving
9 mg	1 clove	3 g	0 mg

Remark: Low oxalate food (Less than 25 mg per serving).

Garlic Powder

Avg Oxalate per 100 g	Serving Size	Serving (g)	Calculated Oxalate per Serving
17 mg	1 tsp	3.1 g	1 mg

Remark: Low oxalate food (Less than 25 mg per serving).

Gatorade

Avg Oxalate per 100 g	Serving Size	Serving (g)	Calculated Oxalate per Serving
0 mg	1 bottle	609 g	0 mg

Remark: Low oxalate food (Less than 25 mg per serving).

Gelatin

Avg Oxalate per 100 g	Serving Size	Serving (g)	Calculated Oxalate per Serving
7 mg	½ cup prepared	22 g	2 mg

Remark: Low oxalate food (Less than 25 mg per serving).

Gin

Avg Oxalate per 100 g	Serving Size	Serving (g)	Calculated Oxalate per Serving
1 mg	1.5 oz	28.4 g	0 mg

Remark: Low oxalate food (Less than 25 mg per serving).

Ginger

Avg Oxalate per 100 g	Serving Size	Serving (g)	Calculated Oxalate per Serving
178 mg	1 tsp sliced	1.8 g	3 mg

Remark: Low oxalate food (Less than 25 mg per serving).

Ginkgo Biloba (Capsule)

Avg Oxalate per 100 g	Serving Size	Serving (g)	Calculated Oxalate per Serving
2034 mg	1 capsule	0.28 g	6 mg

Remark: Low oxalate food (Less than 25 mg per serving).

Ginkgo Nuts

Avg Oxalate per 100 g	Serving Size	Serving (g)	Calculated Oxalate per Serving
26 mg	1 oz	28.35 g	7 mg

Remark: Low oxalate food (Less than 25 mg per serving).

Goat Cheese

Avg Oxalate per 100 g	Serving Size	Serving (g)	Calculated Oxalate per Serving
0 mg	1 oz	28.35 g	0 mg

Remark: Low oxalate food (Less than 25 mg per serving).

Goat Meat

Avg Oxalate per 100 g	Serving Size	Serving (g)	Calculated Oxalate per Serving
0 mg	1 oz	28.35 g	0 mg

Remark: Low oxalate food (Less than 25 mg per serving).

Goat Milk

Avg Oxalate per 100 g	Serving Size	Serving (g)	Calculated Oxalate per Serving
0 mg	1 cup	244 g	0 mg

Remark: Low oxalate food (Less than 25 mg per serving).

Good King Henry (Boiled)

Avg Oxalate per 100 g	Serving Size	Serving (g)	Calculated Oxalate per Serving
245 mg	½ cup	45 g	110 mg

Remark: High oxalate food (100–299 mg per serving).

Good King Henry (Raw)

Avg Oxalate per 100 g	Serving Size	Serving (g)	Calculated Oxalate per Serving
475 mg	½ cup	48 g	228 mg

Remark: High oxalate food (100–299 mg per serving).

Gooseberries

Avg Oxalate per 100 g	Serving Size	Serving (g)	Calculated Oxalate per Serving
22 mg	1 cup	150 g	33 mg

Remark: Moderate oxalate food (25–99 mg per serving).

Gouda Cheese

Avg Oxalate per 100 g	Serving Size	Serving (g)	Calculated Oxalate per Serving
0 mg	1 oz	28.35 g	0 mg

Remark: **Low oxalate food** (Less than 25 mg per serving).

Graham Cracker

Avg Oxalate per 100 g	Serving Size	Serving (g)	Calculated Oxalate per Serving
29 mg	8 crackers	29 g	9 mg

Remark: **Low oxalate food** (Less than 25 mg per serving).

Granola Bars – Hard & Plain

Avg Oxalate per 100 g	Serving Size	Serving (g)	Calculated Oxalate per Serving
18 mg	1 bar	33 g	6 mg

Remark: **Low oxalate food** (Less than 25 mg per serving).

Grape

Avg Oxalate per 100 g	Serving Size	Serving (g)	Calculated Oxalate per Serving
4 mg	1 cup	92 g	3 mg

Remark: Low oxalate food (Less than 25 mg per serving).

Grape Juice

Avg Oxalate per 100 g	Serving Size	Serving (g)	Calculated Oxalate per Serving
1 mg	1 cup	250 g	3 mg

Remark: Low oxalate food (Less than 25 mg per serving).

Grape Leaf

Avg Oxalate per 100 g	Serving Size	Serving (g)	Calculated Oxalate per Serving
135 mg	1 leaf	5 g	7 mg

Remark: Low oxalate food (Less than 25 mg per serving).

Grapefruit

Avg Oxalate per 100 g	Serving Size	Serving (g)	Calculated Oxalate per Serving
11 mg	½ grapefruit (3¼ in diameter)	123 g	13 mg

Remark: **Low oxalate food** (Less than 25 mg per serving).

Grapefruit Juice

Avg Oxalate per 100 g	Serving Size	Serving (g)	Calculated Oxalate per Serving
0 mg	1 cup	250 g	0 mg

Remark: **Low oxalate food** (Less than 25 mg per serving).

Grape-Nuts Flakes (Cereal)

Avg Oxalate per 100 g	Serving Size	Serving (g)	Calculated Oxalate per Serving
57 mg	1 cup	43 g	25 mg

Remark: **Moderate oxalate food** (25–99 mg per serving).

Greek Yogurt

Avg Oxalate per 100 g	Serving Size	Serving (g)	Calculated Oxalate per Serving
0.4 mg	8 oz	227 g	0.8 mg

Remark: Low oxalate food (Less than 25 mg per serving).

Green Beans

Avg Oxalate per 100 g	Serving Size	Serving (g)	Calculated Oxalate per Serving
24 mg	½ cup	62 g	15 mg

Remark: Low oxalate food (Less than 25 mg per serving).

Green Peas

Avg Oxalate per 100 g	Serving Size	Serving (g)	Calculated Oxalate per Serving
26 mg	½ cup	72.5 g	19 mg

Remark: Low oxalate food (Less than 25 mg per serving).

Green Pigeon Peas

Avg Oxalate per 100 g	Serving Size	Serving (g)	Calculated Oxalate per Serving
36 mg	½ cup	31.5 g	11 mg

Remark: Low oxalate food (Less than 25 mg per serving).

Green Tea

Avg Oxalate per 100 g	Serving Size	Serving (g)	Calculated Oxalate per Serving
9 mg	1 cup	240 g	21 mg

Remark: Low oxalate food (Less than 25 mg per serving).

Ground Cloves

Avg Oxalate per 100 g	Serving Size	Serving (g)	Calculated Oxalate per Serving
2001 mg	1 tsp	2.1 g	42 mg

Remark: Moderate oxalate food (25–99 mg per serving).

Ground Flaxseed

Avg Oxalate per 100 g	Serving Size	Serving (g)	Calculated Oxalate per Serving
8 mg	¼ cup	26 g	2 mg

Remark: Low oxalate food (Less than 25 mg per serving).

Ground Ginger

Avg Oxalate per 100 g	Serving Size	Serving (g)	Calculated Oxalate per Serving
38 mg	1 tsp	1.8 g	1 mg

Remark: Low oxalate food (Less than 25 mg per serving).

Gruyere Cheese

Avg Oxalate per 100 g	Serving Size	Serving (g)	Calculated Oxalate per Serving
0 mg	1 oz	28.35 g	0 mg

Remark: Low oxalate food (Less than 25 mg per serving).

Guava

Avg Oxalate per 100 g	Serving Size	Serving (g)	Calculated Oxalate per Serving
70 mg	1 medium	120 g	83 mg

Remark: **Moderate oxalate food** (25–99 mg per serving).

Habanero Pepper

Avg Oxalate per 100 g	Serving Size	Serving (g)	Calculated Oxalate per Serving
11 mg	4 small peppers	14.5 g	2 mg

Remark: **Low oxalate food** (Less than 25 mg per serving).

Haddock

Avg Oxalate per 100 g	Serving Size	Serving (g)	Calculated Oxalate per Serving
0 mg	1 fillet	150 g	0 mg

Remark: **Low oxalate food** (Less than 25 mg per serving).

Ham

Avg Oxalate per 100 g	Serving Size	Serving (g)	Calculated Oxalate per Serving
0.5 mg	1 cup	150 g	1 mg

Remark: Low oxalate food (Less than 25 mg per serving).

Hamburger (Wendy's)

Avg Oxalate per 100 g	Serving Size	Serving (g)	Calculated Oxalate per Serving
11 mg	1 burger	68 g	7 mg

Remark: Low oxalate food (Less than 25 mg per serving).

Hamburger Bun

Avg Oxalate per 100 g	Serving Size	Serving (g)	Calculated Oxalate per Serving
19 mg	1 bun	43 g	8 mg

Remark: Low oxalate food (Less than 25 mg per serving).

Hazelnut

Avg Oxalate per 100 g	Serving Size	Serving (g)	Calculated Oxalate per Serving
181 mg	¼ cup	29 g	53 mg

Remark: **Moderate oxalate food** (25–99 mg per serving).

Hazelnut Milk

Avg Oxalate per 100 g	Serving Size	Serving (g)	Calculated Oxalate per Serving
5 mg	1 cup	242 g	12 mg

Remark: **Low oxalate food (**Less than 25 mg per serving).

Heavily Stuffed Beef Ravioli

Avg Oxalate per 100 g	Serving Size	Serving (g)	Calculated Oxalate per Serving
12 mg	1 cup	260 g	31 mg

Remark: **Moderate oxalate food** (25–99 mg per serving)

Hemp Milk

Avg Oxalate per 100 g	Serving Size	Serving (g)	Calculated Oxalate per Serving
2 mg	1 cup	242 g	5 mg

Remark: Low oxalate food (Less than 25 mg per serving).

Hemp Seeds

Avg Oxalate per 100 g	Serving Size	Serving (g)	Calculated Oxalate per Serving
55 mg	2 tbsp	20 g	11 mg

Remark: Low oxalate food (Less than 25 mg per serving).

Herbal Teas

Avg Oxalate per 100 g	Serving Size	Serving (g)	Calculated Oxalate per Serving
2 mg	1 cup	240 g	5 mg

Remark: Low oxalate food (Less than 25 mg per serving).

Herring

Avg Oxalate per 100 g	Serving Size	Serving (g)	Calculated Oxalate per Serving
0.6 mg	1 fillet	143 g	1 mg

Remark: Low oxalate food (Less than 25 mg per serving).

Hodgson Mill Pasta (Cooked)

Avg Oxalate per 100 g	Serving Size	Serving (g)	Calculated Oxalate per Serving
39 mg	1 cup	144 g	56 mg

Remark: Moderate oxalate food (25–99 mg per serving).

Honey

Avg Oxalate per 100 g	Serving Size	Serving (g)	Calculated Oxalate per Serving
4 mg	1 tbsp	21 g	1 mg

Remark: Low oxalate food (Less than 25 mg per serving).

Honey Toasted Oats (Cereal)

Avg Oxalate per 100 g	Serving Size	Serving (g)	Calculated Oxalate per Serving
63 mg	1 cup	40 g	25 mg

Remark: Moderate oxalate food (25–99 mg per serving).

Honeydew Melon

Avg Oxalate per 100 g	Serving Size	Serving (g)	Calculated Oxalate per Serving
0.7 mg	1 cup	177 g	1 mg

Remark: Low oxalate food (Less than 25 mg per serving).

Horse Meat

Avg Oxalate per 100 g	Serving Size	Serving (g)	Calculated Oxalate per Serving
0 mg	3 oz	85 g	0 mg

Remark: Low oxalate food (Less than 25 mg per serving).

Horseradish

Avg Oxalate per 100 g	Serving Size	Serving (g)	Calculated Oxalate per Serving
13 mg	1 tsp	5 g	1 mg

Remark: **Low oxalate food** (Less than 25 mg per serving).

Hot Chocolate

Avg Oxalate per 100 g	Serving Size	Serving (g)	Calculated Oxalate per Serving
213 mg	3 tbsp	31 g	66 mg

Remark: **Moderate oxalate food** (25–99 mg per serving).

Hotdog (Bread)

Avg Oxalate per 100 g	Serving Size	Serving (g)	Calculated Oxalate per Serving
19 mg	1 bun	43 g	8 mg

Remark: **Low oxalate food** (Less than 25 mg per serving).

Huckleberries

Avg Oxalate per 100 g	Serving Size	Serving (g)	Calculated Oxalate per Serving
47 mg	½ cup	84 g	39 mg

Remark: Moderate oxalate food (25–99 mg per serving).

Hummus

Avg Oxalate per 100 g	Serving Size	Serving (g)	Calculated Oxalate per Serving
13 mg	1 cup	246 g	32 mg

Remark: Moderate oxalate food (25–99 mg per serving).

Ice Cream

Avg Oxalate per 100 g	Serving Size	Serving (g)	Calculated Oxalate per Serving
0 mg	½ cup	76 g	0 mg

Remark: Low oxalate food (Less than 25 mg per serving).

Iced Tea

Avg Oxalate per 100 g	Serving Size	Serving (g)	Calculated Oxalate per Serving
0.3 mg	1 fl oz	30.6 g	0 mg

Remark: Low oxalate food (Less than 25 mg per serving).

Instant Coffee

Avg Oxalate per 100 g	Serving Size	Serving (g)	Calculated Oxalate per Serving
3.2 mg	1 serving (6 fl oz)	179 g	6 mg

Remark: Low oxalate food (Less than 25 mg per serving).

Jalapeño Pepper

Avg Oxalate per 100 g	Serving Size	Serving (g)	Calculated Oxalate per Serving
28 mg	2 small peppers	35 g	10 mg

Remark: Low oxalate food (Less than 25 mg per serving).

Jello

Avg Oxalate per 100 g	Serving Size	Serving (g)	Calculated Oxalate per Serving
7 mg	½ cup prepared	22 g	2 mg

Remark: **Low oxalate food** (Less than 25 mg per serving).

Jicama (Raw)

Avg Oxalate per 100 g	Serving Size	Serving (g)	Calculated Oxalate per Serving
11 mg	1 cup, sliced	120 g	13 mg

Remark: **Low oxalate food** (Less than 25 mg per serving).

Kale (Cooked)

Avg Oxalate per 100 g	Serving Size	Serving (g)	Calculated Oxalate per Serving
5 mg	½ cup	65 g	3 mg

Remark: **Low oxalate food** (Less than 25 mg per serving).

Kefir

Avg Oxalate per 100 g	Serving Size	Serving (g)	Calculated Oxalate per Serving
0 mg	½ cup	122 g	0 mg

Remark: Low oxalate food (Less than 25 mg per serving).

Ketchup

Avg Oxalate per 100 g	Serving Size	Serving (g)	Calculated Oxalate per Serving
8 mg	1 tbsp	15 g	1 mg

Remark: Low oxalate food (Less than 25 mg per serving).

Kidney Beans

Avg Oxalate per 100 g	Serving Size	Serving (g)	Calculated Oxalate per Serving
20 mg	½ cup	109 g	22 mg

Remark: Low oxalate food (Less than 25 mg per serving).

Kiwi

Avg Oxalate per 100 g	Serving Size	Serving (g)	Calculated Oxalate per Serving
36 mg	1 medium (without skin)	76 g	27 mg

Remark: **Moderate oxalate food** (25–99 mg per serving).

Kohlrabi

Avg Oxalate per 100 g	Serving Size	Serving (g)	Calculated Oxalate per Serving
1 mg	1 cup sliced	165 g	1 mg

Remark: **Low oxalate food** (Less than 25 mg per serving)

Lablab

Avg Oxalate per 100 g	Serving Size	Serving (g)	Calculated Oxalate per Serving
25 mg	1 cup	194 g	49 mg

Remark: **Moderate oxalate food** (25–99 mg per serving).

Lamb

Avg Oxalate per 100 g	Serving Size	Serving (g)	Calculated Oxalate per Serving
0 mg	1 oz	85 g	0 mg

Remark: **Low oxalate food** (Less than 25 mg per serving).

Lambsquarters

Avg Oxalate per 100 g	Serving Size	Serving (g)	Calculated Oxalate per Serving
1112 mg	1 cup	26.2 g	289 mg

Remark: **High oxalate food** (100–299 mg per serving).

Lasagna

Avg Oxalate per 100 g	Serving Size	Serving (g)	Calculated Oxalate per Serving
26 mg	1 piece	123 g	32 mg

Remark: **Moderate oxalate food** (25–99 mg per serving).

Leberkäse

Avg Oxalate per 100 g	Serving Size	Serving (g)	Calculated Oxalate per Serving
0 mg	1 oz	28.35 g	0 mg

Remark: Low oxalate food (Less than 25 mg per serving).

Lecithin

Avg Oxalate per 100 g	Serving Size	Serving (g)	Calculated Oxalate per Serving
9 mg	1 tbsp	15 g	1 mg

Remark: Low oxalate food (Less than 25 mg per serving).

Leeks

Avg Oxalate per 100 g	Serving Size	Serving (g)	Calculated Oxalate per Serving
17 mg	1 cup	89 g	15 mg

Remark: Low oxalate food (Less than 25 mg per serving).

Lemon

Avg Oxalate per 100 g	Serving Size	Serving (g)	Calculated Oxalate per Serving
8 mg	1 slice	7 g	1 mg

Remark: Low oxalate food (Less than 25 mg per serving).

Lemon Balm (Leaves)

Avg Oxalate per 100 g	Serving Size	Serving (g)	Calculated Oxalate per Serving
27 mg	¼ cup	20 g	5 mg

Remark: Low oxalate food (Less than 25 mg per serving).

Lemon Juice

Avg Oxalate per 100 g	Serving Size	Serving (g)	Calculated Oxalate per Serving
1 mg	1 cup	244 g	1 mg

Remark: Low oxalate food (Less than 25 mg per serving).

Lemon Myrtle

Avg Oxalate per 100 g	Serving Size	Serving (g)	Calculated Oxalate per Serving
2853 mg	1 tsp	1.7 g	49 mg

Remark: *Moderate oxalate food* (25–99 mg per serving).

Lemon Peel

Avg Oxalate per 100 g	Serving Size	Serving (g)	Calculated Oxalate per Serving
673 mg	1 tsp	2 g	13 mg

Remark: Low oxalate food (Less than 25 mg per serving).

Lemon Tea

Avg Oxalate per 100 g	Serving Size	Serving (g)	Calculated Oxalate per Serving
17 mg	1 cup	266 g	45 mg

Remark: Moderate oxalate food (25–99 mg per serving).

Lemonade

Avg Oxalate per 100 g	Serving Size	Serving (g)	Calculated Oxalate per Serving
6 mg	1 cup (8 fl oz)	247 g	15 mg

Remark: Low oxalate food (Less than 25 mg per serving).

Lentil

Avg Oxalate per 100 g	Serving Size	Serving (g)	Calculated Oxalate per Serving
9 mg	½ cup	96 g	8 mg

Remark: Low oxalate food (Less than 25 mg per serving).

Lime

Avg Oxalate per 100 g	Serving Size	Serving (g)	Calculated Oxalate per Serving
7 mg	1 lime	67 g	4 mg

Remark: Low oxalate food (Less than 25 mg per serving).

Lime Juice

Avg Oxalate per 100 g	Serving Size	Serving (g)	Calculated Oxalate per Serving
2 mg	1 cup	240 g	4 mg

Remark: Low oxalate food (Less than 25 mg per serving).

Liver

Avg Oxalate per 100 g	Serving Size	Serving (g)	Calculated Oxalate per Serving
0 mg	3 oz	85 g	0 mg

Remark: Low oxalate food (Less than 25 mg per serving).

Lotus Seeds

Avg Oxalate per 100 g	Serving Size	Serving (g)	Calculated Oxalate per Serving
66 mg	1 cup	32 g	21 mg

Remark: Low oxalate food (Less than 25 mg per serving).

Macadamia

Avg Oxalate per 100 g	Serving Size	Serving (g)	Calculated Oxalate per Serving
44 mg	¼ cup	29 g	13 mg

Remark: **Low oxalate food** (Less than 25 mg per serving).

Macadamia Milk

Avg Oxalate per 100 g	Serving Size	Serving (g)	Calculated Oxalate per Serving
1 mg	1 cup	242 g	1 mg

Remark: **Low oxalate food** (Less than 25 mg per serving).

Mackerel

Avg Oxalate per 100 g	Serving Size	Serving (g)	Calculated Oxalate per Serving
0 mg	1 fillet	88 g	0 mg

Remark: **Low oxalate food** (Less than 25 mg per serving).

Malt Beer

Avg Oxalate per 100 g	Serving Size	Serving (g)	Calculated Oxalate per Serving
1.78 mg	11.2 fl oz	335 g	3 mg

Remark: Low oxalate food (Less than 25 mg per serving).

Mandarin Orange

Avg Oxalate per 100 g	Serving Size	Serving (g)	Calculated Oxalate per Serving
17 mg	1 medium or ½ cup	82 g	14 mg

Remark: Low oxalate food (Less than 25 mg per serving).

Mango

Avg Oxalate per 100 g	Serving Size	Serving (g)	Calculated Oxalate per Serving
4 mg	1 cup, cubed	165 g	7 mg

Remark: Low oxalate food (Less than 25 mg per serving).

Mango Juice

Avg Oxalate per 100 g	Serving Size	Serving (g)	Calculated Oxalate per Serving
11 mg	1 cup	250 g	27 mg

Remark: **Moderate oxalate food** (25–99 mg per serving).

Mangold (Spinach Beet)

Avg Oxalate per 100 g	Serving Size	Serving (g)	Calculated Oxalate per Serving
874 mg	½ cup	67.5 g	590 mg

Remark: **Very high oxalate food** (300 mg or higher per serving).

Maple Flavoring

Avg Oxalate per 100 g	Serving Size	Serving (g)	Calculated Oxalate per Serving
8 mg	1 tsp	5 g	0 mg

Remark: **Low oxalate food** (Less than 25 mg per serving).

Maple Syrup

Avg Oxalate per 100 g	Serving Size	Serving (g)	Calculated Oxalate per Serving
3 mg	1 tbsp	20 g	1 mg

Remark: Low oxalate food (Less than 25 mg per serving).

Margarine

Avg Oxalate per 100 g	Serving Size	Serving (g)	Calculated Oxalate per Serving
6 mg	1 tbsp	14 g	0 mg

Remark: Low oxalate food (Less than 25 mg per serving).

Marinara Sauce with Pasta

Avg Oxalate per 100 g	Serving Size	Serving (g)	Calculated Oxalate per Serving
11 mg	2 tbsp	30 g	3 mg

Remark: Low oxalate food (Less than 25 mg per serving).

Mayonnaise

Avg Oxalate per 100 g	Serving Size	Serving (g)	Calculated Oxalate per Serving
2 mg	1 tbsp	14 g	0 mg

Remark: Low oxalate food (Less than 25 mg per serving).

Mexican Cheese

Avg Oxalate per 100 g	Serving Size	Serving (g)	Calculated Oxalate per Serving
0 mg	1 cup	132 g	0 mg

Remark: Low oxalate food (Less than 25 mg per serving)

Mexican Mole Sauce (Almond)

Avg Oxalate per 100 g	Serving Size	Serving (g)	Calculated Oxalate per Serving
245 mg	2 tbsp	32 g	78 mg

Remark: Moderate oxalate food (25–99 mg per serving).

Mexican Mole Sauce (Black)

Avg Oxalate per 100 g	Serving Size	Serving (g)	Calculated Oxalate per Serving
12 mg	2 tbsp	32 g	4 mg

Remark: **Low oxalate food** (Less than 25 mg per serving).

Mexican Mole Sauce (Green)

Avg Oxalate per 100 g	Serving Size	Serving (g)	Calculated Oxalate per Serving
147 mg	2 tbsp	32 g	47 mg

Remark: **Moderate oxalate food** (25–99 mg per serving).

Mexican Mole Sauce (Red)

Avg Oxalate per 100 g	Serving Size	Serving (g)	Calculated Oxalate per Serving
321 mg	2 tbsp	32 g	103 mg

Remark: **High oxalate food** (100–299 mg per serving).

Milano Cookies

Avg Oxalate per 100 g	Serving Size	Serving (g)	Calculated Oxalate per Serving
80 mg	2 cookies	27 g	22 mg

Remark: **Low oxalate food (**Less than 25 mg per serving).

Milk Thistle, Seed

Avg Oxalate per 100 g	Serving Size	Serving (g)	Calculated Oxalate per Serving
1517 mg	1 tsp	3 g	46 mg

Remark: **Moderate oxalate food** (25–99 mg per serving)

Milk Thistle, Seed Powder

Avg Oxalate per 100 g	Serving Size	Serving (g)	Calculated Oxalate per Serving
1802 mg	1 tsp	5 g	90 mg

Remark: **Moderate oxalate food** (25–99 mg per serving)

Millet

Avg Oxalate per 100 g	Serving Size	Serving (g)	Calculated Oxalate per Serving
37 mg	½ cup	87 g	32 mg

Remark: **Moderate oxalate food** (25–99 mg per serving).

Miso

Avg Oxalate per 100 g	Serving Size	Serving (g)	Calculated Oxalate per Serving
10 mg	1 tbsp	17 g	2 mg

Remark: **Low oxalate food** (Less than 25 mg per serving).

Mixed Berries Yogurt

Avg Oxalate per 100 g	Serving Size	Serving (g)	Calculated Oxalate per Serving
2 mg	6 oz	170 g	3 mg

Remark: **Low oxalate food** (Less than 25 mg per serving).

Mixed Nuts

Avg Oxalate per 100 g	Serving Size	Serving (g)	Calculated Oxalate per Serving
159 mg	1 cup	134 g	214 mg

Remark: High oxalate food (100–299 mg per serving).

Molasses (Full Flavor)

Avg Oxalate per 100 g	Serving Size	Serving (g)	Calculated Oxalate per Serving
43 mg	1 tbsp	15 g	6 mg

Remark: Low oxalate food (Less than 25 mg per serving).

Mortadella

Avg Oxalate per 100 g	Serving Size	Serving (g)	Calculated Oxalate per Serving
0 mg	1 oz	28.35 g	0 mg

Remark: Low oxalate food (Less than 25 mg per serving).

Mountain Pepper

Avg Oxalate per 100 g	Serving Size	Serving (g)	Calculated Oxalate per Serving
84 mg	1 tsp	2.4 g	2 mg

Remark: Low oxalate food (Less than 25 mg per serving).

Muenster Cheese

Avg Oxalate per 100 g	Serving Size	Serving (g)	Calculated Oxalate per Serving
0 mg	1 oz	28.35 g	0 mg

Remark: Low oxalate food (Less than 25 mg per serving).

Mung Beans

Avg Oxalate per 100 g	Serving Size	Serving (g)	Calculated Oxalate per Serving
3 mg	½ cup	101 g	3 mg

Remark: Low oxalate food (Less than 25 mg per serving).

Mushrooms

Avg Oxalate per 100 g	Serving Size	Serving (g)	Calculated Oxalate per Serving
1 mg	½ cup, sliced	78 g	1 mg

Remark: Low oxalate food (Less than 25 mg per serving).

Mustard

Avg Oxalate per 100 g	Serving Size	Serving (g)	Calculated Oxalate per Serving
5 mg	1 tbsp	15 g	1 mg

Remark: Low oxalate food (Less than 25 mg per serving).

Mustard Greens

Avg Oxalate per 100 g	Serving Size	Serving (g)	Calculated Oxalate per Serving
7 mg	½ cup, chopped	70 g	5 mg

Remark: Low oxalate food (Less than 25 mg per serving)

Mustard Seed

Avg Oxalate per 100 g	Serving Size	Serving (g)	Calculated Oxalate per Serving
29 mg	1 tsp	2 g	1 mg

Remark: Low oxalate food (Less than 25 mg per serving).

Navy Beans

Avg Oxalate per 100 g	Serving Size	Serving (g)	Calculated Oxalate per Serving
56 mg	½ cup	95 g	53 mg

Remark: Moderate oxalate food (25–99 mg per serving).

Nectarine

Avg Oxalate per 100 g	Serving Size	Serving (g)	Calculated Oxalate per Serving
2 mg	1 medium (2½ in diameter)	142 g	2 mg

Remark: Low oxalate food (Less than 25 mg per serving).

Neufchâtel Cheese

Avg Oxalate per 100 g	Serving Size	Serving (g)	Calculated Oxalate per Serving
0.4 mg	1 oz	28.35 g	0.1 mg

Remark: **Low oxalate food** (Less than 25 mg per serving).

New Mexican Pepper

Avg Oxalate per 100 g	Serving Size	Serving (g)	Calculated Oxalate per Serving
48 mg	½ cup, sliced	46 g	22 mg

Remark: **Low oxalate food** (Less than 25 mg per serving).

Noodles (Uncooked)

Avg Oxalate per 100 g	Serving Size	Serving (g)	Calculated Oxalate per Serving
25 mg	1 cup	160 g	40 mg

Remark: **Moderate oxalate food** (25–99 mg per serving).

Nopal or Prickly Pear (Cooked)

Avg Oxalate per 100 g	Serving Size	Serving (g)	Calculated Oxalate per Serving
116 mg	½ cup	75 g	87 mg

Remark: **Moderate oxalate food** (25–99 mg per serving).

Nopal or Prickly Pear (Raw)

Avg Oxalate per 100 g	Serving Size	Serving (g)	Calculated Oxalate per Serving
152 mg	1 cup	149 g	226 mg

Remark: **High oxalate food** (100–299 mg per serving).

Nutmeg

Avg Oxalate per 100 g	Serving Size	Serving (g)	Calculated Oxalate per Serving
244 mg	1 tsp	2.2 g	5 mg

Remark: **Low oxalate food** (Less than 25 mg per serving).

Oat Bran

Avg Oxalate per 100 g	Serving Size	Serving (g)	Calculated Oxalate per Serving
79 mg	¼ cup	28 g	22 mg

Remark: Low oxalate food (Less than 25 mg per serving).

Oat Flour

Avg Oxalate per 100 g	Serving Size	Serving (g)	Calculated Oxalate per Serving
32 mg	¼ cup	24.5 g	8 mg

Remark: Low oxalate food (Less than 25 mg per serving).

Oat Milk

Avg Oxalate per 100 g	Serving Size	Serving (g)	Calculated Oxalate per Serving
5 mg	1 cup	242 g	11 mg

Remark: Low oxalate food (Less than 25 mg per serving).

Oatmeal Cereal

Avg Oxalate per 100 g	Serving Size	Serving (g)	Calculated Oxalate per Serving
9.3 mg	1 cup	234 g	22 mg

Remark: Low oxalate food (Less than 25 mg per serving).

Okra

Avg Oxalate per 100 g	Serving Size	Serving (g)	Calculated Oxalate per Serving
101 mg	½ cup	56 g	56 mg

Remark: Moderate oxalate food (25–99 mg per serving).

Olives

Avg Oxalate per 100 g	Serving Size	Serving (g)	Calculated Oxalate per Serving
50 mg	6 medium olives	23 g	11 mg

Remark: Low oxalate food (Less than 25 mg per serving).

Omelette

Avg Oxalate per 100 g	Serving Size	Serving (g)	Calculated Oxalate per Serving
0 mg	1 large	61 g	0 mg

Remark: Low oxalate food (Less than 25 mg per serving).

Onion

Avg Oxalate per 100 g	Serving Size	Serving (g)	Calculated Oxalate per Serving
5 mg	1 cup, sliced	120 g	6 mg

Remark: Low oxalate food (Less than 25 mg per serving).

Orange

Avg Oxalate per 100 g	Serving Size	Serving (g)	Calculated Oxalate per Serving
13 mg	1 medium	140 g	18 mg

Remark: Low oxalate food (Less than 25 mg per serving).

Orange Extract

Avg Oxalate per 100 g	Serving Size	Serving (g)	Calculated Oxalate per Serving
2 mg	1 tsp	5 g	0 mg

Remark: Low oxalate food (Less than 25 mg per serving).

Oregano

Avg Oxalate per 100 g	Serving Size	Serving (g)	Calculated Oxalate per Serving
417 mg	1 tsp	1.8 g	8 mg

Remark: Low oxalate food (Less than 25 mg per serving).

Ovaltine

Avg Oxalate per 100 g	Serving Size	Serving (g)	Calculated Oxalate per Serving
53 mg	2 tbsp	11 g	6 mg

Remark: Low oxalate food (Less than 25 mg per serving).

Oyster Crackers

Avg Oxalate per 100 g	Serving Size	Serving (g)	Calculated Oxalate per Serving
22 mg	1 oz	28 g	6 mg

Remark: **Low oxalate food** (Less than 25 mg per serving).

Palm Oil

Avg Oxalate per 100 g	Serving Size	Serving (g)	Calculated Oxalate per Serving
0 mg	1 tbsp	14 g	0 mg

Remark: **Low oxalate food** (Less than 25 mg per serving).

Pancake Mix

Avg Oxalate per 100 g	Serving Size	Serving (g)	Calculated Oxalate per Serving
23 mg	¼ cup, dry	30 g	7 mg

Remark: **Low oxalate food** (Less than 25 mg per serving).

Pancakes (Homemade)

Avg Oxalate per 100 g	Serving Size	Serving (g)	Calculated Oxalate per Serving
12.8 mg	1 pancake	28.35 g	4 mg

Remark: **Low oxalate food** (Less than 25 mg per serving).

Papaya

Avg Oxalate per 100 g	Serving Size	Serving (g)	Calculated Oxalate per Serving
1 mg	½ cup, mashed	115 g	1 mg

Remark: **Low oxalate food** (Less than 25 mg per serving).

Papaya Seed

Avg Oxalate per 100 g	Serving Size	Serving (g)	Calculated Oxalate per Serving
154 mg	2 tbsp	20 g	31 mg

Remark: **Moderate oxalate food** (25–99 mg per serving).

Paprika

Avg Oxalate per 100 g	Serving Size	Serving (g)	Calculated Oxalate per Serving
284 mg	1 tsp	2.1 g	6 mg

Remark: Low oxalate food (Less than 25 mg per serving).

Parmigiano-Reggiano

Avg Oxalate per 100 g	Serving Size	Serving (g)	Calculated Oxalate per Serving
0 mg	1 oz	28.35 g	0 mg

Remark: Low oxalate food (Less than 25 mg per serving).

Parsnips

Avg Oxalate per 100 g	Serving Size	Serving (g)	Calculated Oxalate per Serving
19 mg	½ cup, sliced	78 g	15 mg

Remark: Low oxalate food (Less than 25 mg per serving).

Pasilla Chili

Avg Oxalate per 100 g	Serving Size	Serving (g)	Calculated Oxalate per Serving
103 mg	1 tsp	2 g	2 mg

Remark: Low oxalate food (Less than 25 mg per serving).

Passion Fruit or Granadilla

Avg Oxalate per 100 g	Serving Size	Serving (g)	Calculated Oxalate per Serving
1 mg	1 passion fruit	18 g	0 mg

Remark: Low oxalate food (Less than 25 mg per serving).

Pasta (Non-Whole Wheat Varieties)

Avg Oxalate per 100 g	Serving Size	Serving (g)	Calculated Oxalate per Serving
18 mg	1 cup	128 g	24 mg

Remark: Low oxalate food (Less than 25 mg per serving).

Pasta (Whole Wheat Varieties)

Avg Oxalate per 100 g	Serving Size	Serving (g)	Calculated Oxalate per Serving
25 mg	1 cup	128 g	31 mg

Remark: **Moderate oxalate food** (25–99 mg per serving).

Pea Milk

Avg Oxalate per 100 g	Serving Size	Serving (g)	Calculated Oxalate per Serving
0 mg	1 cup	242 g	0 mg

Remark: **Low oxalate food** (Less than 25 mg per serving).

Peach (Canned)

Avg Oxalate per 100 g	Serving Size	Serving (g)	Calculated Oxalate per Serving
2 mg	1 small or ½ cup sliced	127 g	3 mg

Remark: **Low oxalate food** (Less than 25 mg per serving).

Peanut Butter

Avg Oxalate per 100 g	Serving Size	Serving (g)	Calculated Oxalate per Serving
125 mg	2 tbsp	29 g	36 mg

Remark: Moderate oxalate food (25–99 mg per serving).

Peanut Butter Bar

Avg Oxalate per 100 g	Serving Size	Serving (g)	Calculated Oxalate per Serving
106 mg	1 bar	68 g	72 mg

Remark: Moderate oxalate food (25–99 mg per serving).

Peanut Candy

Avg Oxalate per 100 g	Serving Size	Serving (g)	Calculated Oxalate per Serving
46 mg	10 pieces	24 g	11 mg

Remark: Low oxalate food (Less than 25 mg per serving).

Peanut Oil

Avg Oxalate per 100 g	Serving Size	Serving (g)	Calculated Oxalate per Serving
418 mg	1 tbsp	13.5 g	56 mg

Remark: **Moderate oxalate food** (25–99 mg per serving).

Peanuts

Avg Oxalate per 100 g	Serving Size	Serving (g)	Calculated Oxalate per Serving
131 mg	¼ cup	29 g	38 mg

Remark: **Moderate oxalate food** (25–99 mg per serving).

Pear

Avg Oxalate per 100 g	Serving Size	Serving (g)	Calculated Oxalate per Serving
5 mg	½ cup	84 g	4 mg

Remark: **Low oxalate food** (Less than 25 mg per serving).

Pecans

Avg Oxalate per 100 g	Serving Size	Serving (g)	Calculated Oxalate per Serving
52 mg	¼ cup	29 g	15 mg

Remark: Low oxalate food (Less than 25 mg per serving).

Peppermint Leaves

Avg Oxalate per 100 g	Serving Size	Serving (g)	Calculated Oxalate per Serving
56 mg	2 leaves	0.1 g	0 mg

Remark: Low oxalate food (Less than 25 mg per serving).

Pepperoni

Avg Oxalate per 100 g	Serving Size	Serving (g)	Calculated Oxalate per Serving
0 mg	3 oz	85 g	0 mg

Remark: Low oxalate food (Less than 25 mg per serving).

Peppers (Sweet and Hot, Variety)

Avg Oxalate per 100 g	Serving Size	Serving (g)	Calculated Oxalate per Serving
20 mg	½ cup, sliced	57 g	11 mg

Remark: **Low oxalate food** (Less than 25 mg per serving).

Persimmons (Hachiya)

Avg Oxalate per 100 g	Serving Size	Serving (g)	Calculated Oxalate per Serving
9 mg	1 medium	200 g	19 mg

Remark: **Low oxalate food** (Less than 25 mg per serving).

Pickles

Avg Oxalate per 100 g	Serving Size	Serving (g)	Calculated Oxalate per Serving
9 mg	1 pickle	28 g	3 mg

Remark: **Low oxalate food** (Less than 25 mg per serving).

Pie Crust

Avg Oxalate per 100 g	Serving Size	Serving (g)	Calculated Oxalate per Serving
24 mg	⅛ crust	19.5 g	5 mg

Remark: Low oxalate food (Less than 25 mg per serving).

Pili Nuts

Avg Oxalate per 100 g	Serving Size	Serving (g)	Calculated Oxalate per Serving
1 mg	1 cup	120 g	1 mg

Remark: Low oxalate food (Less than 25 mg per serving).

Pine Nuts

Avg Oxalate per 100 g	Serving Size	Serving (g)	Calculated Oxalate per Serving
185 mg	¼ cup	29 g	54 mg

Remark: Moderate oxalate food (25–99 mg per serving).

Pineapple

Avg Oxalate per 100 g	Serving Size	Serving (g)	Calculated Oxalate per Serving
6 mg	½ cup	112 g	7 mg

Remark: Low oxalate food (Less than 25 mg per serving).

Pineapple Juice

Avg Oxalate per 100 g	Serving Size	Serving (g)	Calculated Oxalate per Serving
1 mg	1 cup	250 g	2 mg

Remark: Low oxalate food (Less than 25 mg per serving).

Pinto Beans

Avg Oxalate per 100 g	Serving Size	Serving (g)	Calculated Oxalate per Serving
34 mg	½ cup	85 g	29 mg

Remark: Moderate oxalate food (25–99 mg per serving).

Pistachio

Avg Oxalate per 100 g	Serving Size	Serving (g)	Calculated Oxalate per Serving
42 mg	¼ cup	29 g	12 mg

Remark: Low oxalate food (Less than 25 mg per serving).

Pizza Crust

Avg Oxalate per 100 g	Serving Size	Serving (g)	Calculated Oxalate per Serving
15 mg	½ of 8 in. shell	71 g	11 mg

Remark: Low oxalate food (Less than 25 mg per serving).

Plain Yogurt

Avg Oxalate per 100 g	Serving Size	Serving (g)	Calculated Oxalate per Serving
0.3 mg	1 can	0.3 g	1 mg

Remark: Low oxalate food (Less than 25 mg per serving).

Plantain

Avg Oxalate per 100 g	Serving Size	Serving (g)	Calculated Oxalate per Serving
0.5 mg	1 plantain	200 g	1 mg

Remark: Low oxalate food (Less than 25 mg per serving).

Plantain Chips

Avg Oxalate per 100 g	Serving Size	Serving (g)	Calculated Oxalate per Serving
3 mg	1 oz	28 g	1 mg

Remark: Low oxalate food (Less than 25 mg per serving).

Plum Juice

Avg Oxalate per 100 g	Serving Size	Serving (g)	Calculated Oxalate per Serving
3 mg	1 cup	250 g	9 mg

Remark: Low oxalate food (Less than 25 mg per serving).

Plums

Avg Oxalate per 100 g	Serving Size	Serving (g)	Calculated Oxalate per Serving
23 mg	1 cup, sliced	165 g	38 mg

Remark: **Moderate oxalate food** (25–99 mg per serving).

Pomegranate Juice

Avg Oxalate per 100 g	Serving Size	Serving (g)	Calculated Oxalate per Serving
3 mg	1 cup	240 g	8 mg

Remark: **Low oxalate food** (Less than 25 mg per serving).

Pomegranates

Avg Oxalate per 100 g	Serving Size	Serving (g)	Calculated Oxalate per Serving
78 mg	½ medium (4 in. diameter)	141 g	110 mg

Remark: **High oxalate food** (100–299 mg per serving)

Pomelo

Avg Oxalate per 100 g	Serving Size	Serving (g)	Calculated Oxalate per Serving
0 mg	1 cup	190 g	0 mg

Remark: Low oxalate food (Less than 25 mg per serving).

Poppy Seeds

Avg Oxalate per 100 g	Serving Size	Serving (g)	Calculated Oxalate per Serving
1620 mg	1 tsp	2.8 g	45 mg

Remark: Moderate oxalate food (25–99 mg per serving).

Poptart

Avg Oxalate per 100 g	Serving Size	Serving (g)	Calculated Oxalate per Serving
13 mg	1 pastry	52 g	7 mg

Remark: Low oxalate food (Less than 25 mg per serving).

Pork

Avg Oxalate per 100 g	Serving Size	Serving (g)	Calculated Oxalate per Serving
0 mg	3 oz	85 g	0 mg

Remark: Low oxalate food (Less than 25 mg per serving).

Potato (Baked)

Avg Oxalate per 100 g	Serving Size	Serving (g)	Calculated Oxalate per Serving
46 mg	½ cup, chopped	64 g	29 mg

Remark: Moderate oxalate food (25–99 mg per serving).

Potato (White or Red, Boiled)

Avg Oxalate per 100 g	Serving Size	Serving (g)	Calculated Oxalate per Serving
13 mg	½ cup	78 g	10 mg

Remark: Low oxalate food (Less than 25 mg per serving).

Potato (White, Deep Fried)

Avg Oxalate per 100 g	Serving Size	Serving (g)	Calculated Oxalate per Serving
32 mg	½ cup	112 g	36 mg

Remark: **Moderate oxalate food** (25–99 mg per serving).

Potato Chips

Avg Oxalate per 100 g	Serving Size	Serving (g)	Calculated Oxalate per Serving
47 mg	1 oz	28.35 g	13 mg

Remark: **Low oxalate food** (Less than 25 mg per serving).

Potato Flakes

Avg Oxalate per 100 g	Serving Size	Serving (g)	Calculated Oxalate per Serving
12 mg	⅓ cup flakes	17 g	2 mg

Remark: **Low oxalate food** (Less than 25 mg per serving).

Potato Flour

Avg Oxalate per 100 g	Serving Size	Serving (g)	Calculated Oxalate per Serving
3 mg	¼ cup	42 g	1 mg

Remark: Low oxalate food (Less than 25 mg per serving).

Potato Salad

Avg Oxalate per 100 g	Serving Size	Serving (g)	Calculated Oxalate per Serving
19 mg	½ cup	138 g	26 mg

Remark: Moderate oxalate food (25–99 mg per serving).

Powerade

Avg Oxalate per 100 g	Serving Size	Serving (g)	Calculated Oxalate per Serving
0 mg	8 fl oz	244 g	0 mg

Remark: Low oxalate food (Less than 25 mg per serving).

Pretzels Crackers

Avg Oxalate per 100 g	Serving Size	Serving (g)	Calculated Oxalate per Serving
3 mg	14 crackers	28 g	1 mg

Remark: **Low oxalate food** (Less than 25 mg per serving).

Prunes

Avg Oxalate per 100 g	Serving Size	Serving (g)	Calculated Oxalate per Serving
45 mg	¼ cup	66 g	30 mg

Remark: **Moderate oxalate food** (25–99 mg per serving).

Pumpkin

Avg Oxalate per 100 g	Serving Size	Serving (g)	Calculated Oxalate per Serving
6 mg	½ cup	120 g	7 mg

Remark: **Low oxalate food** (Less than 25 mg per serving).

Pumpkin Leaf

Avg Oxalate per 100 g	Serving Size	Serving (g)	Calculated Oxalate per Serving
1 mg	1 cup	39 g	0 mg

Remark: **Low oxalate food** (Less than 25 mg per serving).

Pumpkin Seed

Avg Oxalate per 100 g	Serving Size	Serving (g)	Calculated Oxalate per Serving
9 mg	2 tbsp	20 g	2 mg

Remark: **Low oxalate food** (Less than 25 mg per serving).

Purslane Leaves

Avg Oxalate per 100 g	Serving Size	Serving (g)	Calculated Oxalate per Serving
621 mg	1 cup	40 g	248 mg

Remark: **High oxalate food** (100–299 mg per serving).

Quail

Avg Oxalate per 100 g	Serving Size	Serving (g)	Calculated Oxalate per Serving
0 mg	1 quail	109 g	0 mg

Remark: **Low oxalate food** (Less than 25 mg per serving).

Quinoa (Cooked)

Avg Oxalate per 100 g	Serving Size	Serving (g)	Calculated Oxalate per Serving
61 mg	½ cup, cooked	90 g	55 mg

Remark: **Moderate oxalate food** (25–99 mg per serving).

Quinoa (Raw)

Avg Oxalate per 100 g	Serving Size	Serving (g)	Calculated Oxalate per Serving
106 mg	1 cup	185 g	196 mg

Remark: **High oxalate food** (100–299 mg per serving).

Radish

Avg Oxalate per 100 g	Serving Size	Serving (g)	Calculated Oxalate per Serving
1 mg	1 cup, sliced	100 g	1 mg

Remark: Low oxalate food (Less than 25 mg per serving).

Raspberries

Avg Oxalate per 100 g	Serving Size	Serving (g)	Calculated Oxalate per Serving
17 mg	1 cup	123 g	21 mg

Remark: Low oxalate food (Less than 25 mg per serving).

Ravioli

Avg Oxalate per 100 g	Serving Size	Serving (g)	Calculated Oxalate per Serving
10 mg	1 cup	244 g	25 mg

Remark: Moderate oxalate food (25–99 mg per serving).

Red Cabbage

Avg Oxalate per 100 g	Serving Size	Serving (g)	Calculated Oxalate per Serving
19 mg	1 cup, shredded	70 g	13 mg

Remark: **Low oxalate food** (Less than 25 mg per serving).

Red Currant Juice

Avg Oxalate per 100 g	Serving Size	Serving (g)	Calculated Oxalate per Serving
20 mg	1 cup	112 g	22 mg

Remark: **Low oxalate food** (Less than 25 mg per serving).

Red Wine

Avg Oxalate per 100 g	Serving Size	Serving (g)	Calculated Oxalate per Serving
0 mg	4 oz	112 g	0 mg

Remark: Low oxalate food (Less than 25 mg per serving).

Refried Beans

Avg Oxalate per 100 g	Serving Size	Serving (g)	Calculated Oxalate per Serving
227 mg	1 cup	238 g	540 mg

Remark: **Very high oxalate food** (300 mg or higher per serving).

Rhubarb

Avg Oxalate per 100 g	Serving Size	Serving (g)	Calculated Oxalate per Serving
1060 mg	1 cup, diced	122 g	1293 mg

Remark: **Very high oxalate food** (300 mg or higher per serving).

Rhubarb Juice

Avg Oxalate per 100 g	Serving Size	Serving (g)	Calculated Oxalate per Serving
198 mg	1 cup	250 g	496 mg

Remark: **Very high oxalate food** (300 mg or higher per serving).

Rice (White)

Avg Oxalate per 100 g	Serving Size	Serving (g)	Calculated Oxalate per Serving
4 mg	1 cup	158 g	6 mg

Remark: Low oxalate food (Less than 25 mg per serving).

Rice Cakes (Cracker)

Avg Oxalate per 100 g	Serving Size	Serving (g)	Calculated Oxalate per Serving
31 mg	1 oz	28 g	9 mg

Remark: **Low oxalate food** (Less than 25 mg per serving).

Rice Milk

Avg Oxalate per 100 g	Serving Size	Serving (g)	Calculated Oxalate per Serving
3 mg	1 cup	242 g	7 mg

Remark: **Low oxalate food** (Less than 25 mg per serving).

Ricotta

Avg Oxalate per 100 g	Serving Size	Serving (g)	Calculated Oxalate per Serving
0 mg	1 cup	55 g	0 mg

Remark: Low oxalate food (Less than 25 mg per serving).

Rockfish

Avg Oxalate per 100 g	Serving Size	Serving (g)	Calculated Oxalate per Serving
0 mg	1 fillet	149 g	0 mg

Remark: Low oxalate food (Less than 25 mg per serving).

Romano Cheese

Avg Oxalate per 100 g	Serving Size	Serving (g)	Calculated Oxalate per Serving
0 mg	1 oz	28.35 g	0 mg

Remark: Low oxalate food (Less than 25 mg per serving).

Rosemary

Avg Oxalate per 100 g	Serving Size	Serving (g)	Calculated Oxalate per Serving
219 mg	1 tbsp	2 g	4 mg

Remark: Low oxalate food (Less than 25 mg per serving).

Rum

Avg Oxalate per 100 g	Serving Size	Serving (g)	Calculated Oxalate per Serving
1 mg	1.5 oz	28.4 g	0 mg

Remark: Low oxalate food (Less than 25 mg per serving).

Rutabaga (Raw)

Avg Oxalate per 100 g	Serving Size	Serving (g)	Calculated Oxalate per Serving
30 mg	1 medium	386 g	116 mg

Remark: High oxalate food (100–299 mg per serving).

Rutabaga (Boiled)

Avg Oxalate per 100 g	Serving Size	Serving (g)	Calculated Oxalate per Serving
4 mg	½ cup, cubed	85 g	4 mg

Remark: **Low oxalate food** (Less than 25 mg per serving).

Rye Bread

Avg Oxalate per 100 g	Serving Size	Serving (g)	Calculated Oxalate per Serving
44 mg	1 slice	30 g	13 mg

Remark: **Low oxalate food** (Less than 25 mg per serving).

Rye Crackers

Avg Oxalate per 100 g	Serving Size	Serving (g)	Calculated Oxalate per Serving
55 mg	1 oz	28 g	16 mg

Remark: **Low oxalate food** (Less than 25 mg per serving).

Saccharin

Avg Oxalate per 100 g	Serving Size	Serving (g)	Calculated Oxalate per Serving
5 mg	1 tsp	5 g	0 mg

Remark: Low oxalate food (Less than 25 mg per serving).

Sage

Avg Oxalate per 100 g	Serving Size	Serving (g)	Calculated Oxalate per Serving
574 mg	1 tsp	0.7 g	4 mg

Remark: Low oxalate food (Less than 25 mg per serving).

Salad Dressing

Avg Oxalate per 100 g	Serving Size	Serving (g)	Calculated Oxalate per Serving
5 mg	2 tbsp	30 g	1 mg

Remark: Low oxalate food (Less than 25 mg per serving).

Salami

Avg Oxalate per 100 g	Serving Size	Serving (g)	Calculated Oxalate per Serving
0 mg	1 slice	12.3 g	0 mg

Remark: Low oxalate food (Less than 25 mg per serving).

Salisbury Steak

Avg Oxalate per 100 g	Serving Size	Serving (g)	Calculated Oxalate per Serving
0 mg	1 patty	63 g	0 mg

Remark: Low oxalate food (Less than 25 mg per serving).

Salmon

Avg Oxalate per 100 g	Serving Size	Serving (g)	Calculated Oxalate per Serving
0.2 mg	3 oz	85 g	0 mg

Remark: Low oxalate food (Less than 25 mg per serving).

Saltines Crackers

Avg Oxalate per 100 g	Serving Size	Serving (g)	Calculated Oxalate per Serving
39 mg	3 crackers	15 g	6 mg

Remark: Low oxalate food (Less than 25 mg per serving).

Sandwich (with Spinach)

Avg Oxalate per 100 g	Serving Size	Serving (g)	Calculated Oxalate per Serving
80 mg	1 item	109 g	88 mg

Remark: Moderate oxalate food (25–99 mg per serving).

Sandwich (without Spinach)

Avg Oxalate per 100 g	Serving Size	Serving (g)	Calculated Oxalate per Serving
16 mg	1 item	115 g	18 mg

Remark: Low oxalate food (Less than 25 mg per serving).

Sardine

Avg Oxalate per 100 g	Serving Size	Serving (g)	Calculated Oxalate per Serving
0.3 mg	1 oz	28.35 g	0 mg

Remark: Low oxalate food (Less than 25 mg per serving).

Sauerkraut

Avg Oxalate per 100 g	Serving Size	Serving (g)	Calculated Oxalate per Serving
7 mg	1 cup	142 g	10 mg

Remark: Low oxalate food (Less than 25 mg per serving).

Sausage

Avg Oxalate per 100 g	Serving Size	Serving (g)	Calculated Oxalate per Serving
4 mg	4 oz	113 g	5 mg

Remark: Low oxalate food (Less than 25 mg per serving).

Sausage Biscuit (McDonald's)

Avg Oxalate per 100 g	Serving Size	Serving (g)	Calculated Oxalate per Serving
18 mg	1 biscuit	108 g	20 mg

Remark: **Low oxalate food** (Less than 25 mg per serving).

Sausage McMuffin (McDonald's)

Avg Oxalate per 100 g	Serving Size	Serving (g)	Calculated Oxalate per Serving
18 mg	1 McMuffin	119 g	22 mg

Remark: **Low oxalate food** (Less than 25 mg per serving).

Saviseed

Avg Oxalate per 100 g	Serving Size	Serving (g)	Calculated Oxalate per Serving
247 mg	¼ cup	29 g	72 mg

Remark: **Moderate oxalate food** (25–99 mg per serving).

Savory

Avg Oxalate per 100 g	Serving Size	Serving (g)	Calculated Oxalate per Serving
55 mg	1 tsp	1.4 g	1 mg

Remark: **Low oxalate food** (Less than 25 mg per serving).

Savoy Cabbage

Avg Oxalate per 100 g	Serving Size	Serving (g)	Calculated Oxalate per Serving
4 mg	1 cup, shredded	70 g	3 mg

Remark: **Low oxalate food** (Less than 25 mg per serving).

Scallions

Avg Oxalate per 100 g	Serving Size	Serving (g)	Calculated Oxalate per Serving
7 mg	1 tbsp (chopped)	6 g	0 mg

Remark: **Low oxalate food** (Less than 25 mg per serving).

Scrambled Egg

Avg Oxalate per 100 g	Serving Size	Serving (g)	Calculated Oxalate per Serving
0 mg	2 eggs	96 g	0 mg

Remark: **Low oxalate food** (Less than 25 mg per serving).

Seaweed (Kombu)

Avg Oxalate per 100 g	Serving Size	Serving (g)	Calculated Oxalate per Serving
5 mg	One 1×4 inch piece	4 g	0 mg

Remark: **Low oxalate food** (Less than 25 mg per serving).

Seasoned Salt

Avg Oxalate per 100 g	Serving Size	Serving (g)	Calculated Oxalate per Serving
33 mg	1 tsp	4.8 g	2 mg

Remark: **Low oxalate food** (Less than 25 mg per serving).

Semolina Flour

Avg Oxalate per 100 g	Serving Size	Serving (g)	Calculated Oxalate per Serving
46 mg	¼ cup	41.5 g	19 mg

Remark: Low oxalate food (Less than 25 mg per serving).

Serrano Pepper

Avg Oxalate per 100 g	Serving Size	Serving (g)	Calculated Oxalate per Serving
30 mg	2 small peppers	18 g	5 mg

Remark: Low oxalate food (Less than 25 mg per serving).

Sesame Crackers

Avg Oxalate per 100 g	Serving Size	Serving (g)	Calculated Oxalate per Serving
122 mg	1 oz	28 g	34 mg

Remark: Moderate oxalate food (25–99 mg per serving).

Sesame Seeds (Toasted)

Avg Oxalate per 100 g	Serving Size	Serving (g)	Calculated Oxalate per Serving
216 mg	1 tsp	3 g	6 mg

Remark: **Low oxalate food** (Less than 25 mg per serving).

Sesame Seeds (Whole Dried)

Avg Oxalate per 100 g	Serving Size	Serving (g)	Calculated Oxalate per Serving
3800 mg	1 tsp	3 g	114 mg

Remark: **High oxalate food** (100–299 mg per serving).

Sesame Wheat Crackers

Avg Oxalate per 100 g	Serving Size	Serving (g)	Calculated Oxalate per Serving
384 mg	8 crackers	30 g	115 mg

Remark: **High oxalate food** (100–299 mg per serving).

Shallots

Avg Oxalate per 100 g	Serving Size	Serving (g)	Calculated Oxalate per Serving
2 mg	½ cup, chopped	40 g	1 mg

Remark: **Low oxalate food** (Less than 25 mg per serving).

Sherbet

Avg Oxalate per 100 g	Serving Size	Serving (g)	Calculated Oxalate per Serving
0 mg	1 bar (2.75 fl oz)	66 g	0 mg

Remark: **Low oxalate food** (Less than 25 mg per serving).

Shrimp

Avg Oxalate per 100 g	Serving Size	Serving (g)	Calculated Oxalate per Serving
0.1 mg	3 oz	85 g	0 mg

Remark: **Low oxalate food** (Less than 25 mg per serving).

Shortcake

Avg Oxalate per 100 g	Serving Size	Serving (g)	Calculated Oxalate per Serving
7 mg	1 oz	28.35 g	0 mg

Remark: Low oxalate food (Less than 25 mg per serving).

Snapper

Avg Oxalate per 100 g	Serving Size	Serving (g)	Calculated Oxalate per Serving
0 mg	1 fillet	170 g	0 mg

Remark: Low oxalate food (Less than 25 mg per serving).

Soy Flour

Avg Oxalate per 100 g	Serving Size	Serving (g)	Calculated Oxalate per Serving
135 mg	¼ cup	21 g	28 mg

Remark: Moderate oxalate food (25–99 mg per serving).

Soy Milk

Avg Oxalate per 100 g	Serving Size	Serving (g)	Calculated Oxalate per Serving
4 mg	1 cup	242 g	9 mg

Remark: Low oxalate food (Less than 25 mg per serving).

Soy Sauce

Avg Oxalate per 100 g	Serving Size	Serving (g)	Calculated Oxalate per Serving
9 mg	1 tbsp	15 g	1 mg

Remark: Low oxalate food (Less than 25 mg per serving).

Soybean

Avg Oxalate per 100 g	Serving Size	Serving (g)	Calculated Oxalate per Serving
45 mg	½ cup	86 g	39 mg

Remark: Moderate oxalate food (25–99 mg per serving).

Soybean Crackers

Avg Oxalate per 100 g	Serving Size	Serving (g)	Calculated Oxalate per Serving
204 mg	1 oz	28 g	57 mg

Remark: moderate oxalate food (25–99 mg per serving).

Soynuts

Avg Oxalate per 100 g	Serving Size	Serving (g)	Calculated Oxalate per Serving
84 mg	¼ cup	29 g	24 mg

Remark: Low oxalate food (Less than 25 mg per serving).

Soy Cheese

Avg Oxalate per 100 g	Serving Size	Serving (g)	Calculated Oxalate per Serving
57 mg	1 oz	28 g	16 mg

Remark: Low oxalate food (Less than 25 mg per serving).

Spaghetti

Avg Oxalate per 100 g	Serving Size	Serving (g)	Calculated Oxalate per Serving
13.3 mg	1 cup spaghetti (packed)	150 g	20 mg

Remark: **Low oxalate food** (Less than 25 mg per serving).

Spinach (Raw and Cooked)

Avg Oxalate per 100 g	Serving Size	Serving (g)	Calculated Oxalate per Serving
567 mg	½ cup	87 g	493 mg

Remark: **Very high oxalate food** (300 mg or higher per serving).

Squash

Avg Oxalate per 100 g	Serving Size	Serving (g)	Calculated Oxalate per Serving
4 mg	1 cup, sliced	150 g	6 mg

Remark: **Low oxalate food** (Less than 25 mg per serving).

Star Fruit Juice (Sweet or Sour)

Avg Oxalate per 100 g	Serving Size	Serving (g)	Calculated Oxalate per Serving
829 mg	1 cup	240 g	1990 mg

Remark: **Very high oxalate food** (300 mg or higher per serving).

Stone-ground 7 Grain Crackers, Kashi

Avg Oxalate per 100 g	Serving Size	Serving (g)	Calculated Oxalate per Serving
270 mg	4 crackers	28 g	76 mg

Remark: **moderate oxalate food** (25–99 mg per serving).

Strawberries

Avg Oxalate per 100 g	Serving Size	Serving (g)	Calculated Oxalate per Serving
4 mg	1 cup, halves	150 g	6 mg

Remark: **Low oxalate food** (Less than 25 mg per serving).

Strawberry Yogurt

Avg Oxalate per 100 g	Serving Size	Serving (g)	Calculated Oxalate per Serving
0 mg	6 oz	170 g	1 mg

Remark: Low oxalate food (Less than 25 mg per serving).

Sugar (White)

Avg Oxalate per 100 g	Serving Size	Serving (g)	Calculated Oxalate per Serving
3 mg	1 tsp	4.2 g	0 mg

Remark: Low oxalate food (Less than 25 mg per serving).

Sugar (Brown)

Avg Oxalate per 100 g	Serving Size	Serving (g)	Calculated Oxalate per Serving
11 mg	1 tsp	4.6 g	1 mg

Remark: Low oxalate food (Less than 25 mg per serving).

Sugar Snap

Avg Oxalate per 100 g	Serving Size	Serving (g)	Calculated Oxalate per Serving
32 mg	½ cup	80 g	26 mg

Remark: **Moderate oxalate food** (25–99 mg per serving).

Sunflower Seed

Avg Oxalate per 100 g	Serving Size	Serving (g)	Calculated Oxalate per Serving
22 mg	2 Tbsp	29 g	6 mg

Remark: **Low oxalate food** (Less than 25 mg per serving).

Sweet Potato (With Skin)

Avg Oxalate per 100 g	Serving Size	Serving (g)	Calculated Oxalate per Serving
126 mg	½ cup	125 g	158 mg

Remark: **High oxalate food** (100–299 mg per serving).

Sweet Potato (Without Skin)

Avg Oxalate per 100 g	Serving Size	Serving (g)	Calculated Oxalate per Serving
42 mg	½ cup, mashed	134 g	56 mg

Remark: Moderate oxalate food (25–99 mg per serving).

Sweet Potato Chips

Avg Oxalate per 100 g	Serving Size	Serving (g)	Calculated Oxalate per Serving
219 mg	1 oz	17 g	37 mg

Remark: Moderate oxalate food (25–99 mg per serving).

Sweet Potato Leaves

Avg Oxalate per 100 g	Serving Size	Serving (g)	Calculated Oxalate per Serving
58 mg	1 cup, chopped	36 g	20 mg

Remark: Low oxalate food (Less than 25 mg per serving).

Sweet Potato Soup

Avg Oxalate per 100 g	Serving Size	Serving (g)	Calculated Oxalate per Serving
16 mg	1 cup	245 g	40 mg

Remark: **Moderate oxalate food** (25–99 mg per serving).

Swiss Chard (Boiled and Raw)

Avg Oxalate per 100 g	Serving Size	Serving (g)	Calculated Oxalate per Serving
679 mg	½ cup, chopped	87.5 g	594 mg

Remark: **Very high oxalate food** (300 mg or higher per serving).

Swiss Cheese

Avg Oxalate per 100 g	Serving Size	Serving (g)	Calculated Oxalate per Serving
0 mg	1 oz	28.35 g	0 mg

Remark: **Low oxalate food** (Less than 25 mg per serving).

Tabasco Pepper

Avg Oxalate per 100 g	Serving Size	Serving (g)	Calculated Oxalate per Serving
3 mg	2 small peppers	18.5 g	1 mg

Remark: Low oxalate food (Less than 25 mg per serving).

Taro Leaves

Avg Oxalate per 100 g	Serving Size	Serving (g)	Calculated Oxalate per Serving
652 mg	1 cup	28 g	183 mg

Remark: High oxalate food (100–299 mg per serving).

Tarragon

Avg Oxalate per 100 g	Serving Size	Serving (g)	Calculated Oxalate per Serving
118 mg	1 tsp	1.6 g	2 mg

Remark: Low oxalate food (Less than 25 mg per serving).

Tequila

Avg Oxalate per 100 g	Serving Size	Serving (g)	Calculated Oxalate per Serving
1 mg	1.5 oz	28.4 g	0 mg

Remark: Low oxalate food (Less than 25 mg per serving).

Thyme

Avg Oxalate per 100 g	Serving Size	Serving (g)	Calculated Oxalate per Serving
182 mg	1 tsp	1.4 g	3 mg

Remark: Low oxalate food (Less than 25 mg per serving).

Tigernut Flour

Avg Oxalate per 100 g	Serving Size	Serving (g)	Calculated Oxalate per Serving
41 mg	¼ cup	30 g	12 mg

Remark: Low oxalate food (Less than 25 mg per serving).

Tofu

Avg Oxalate per 100 g	Serving Size	Serving (g)	Calculated Oxalate per Serving
8 mg	½ cup, cubed	125 g	10 mg

Remark: Low oxalate food (Less than 25 mg per serving).

Tomatillo

Avg Oxalate per 100 g	Serving Size	Serving (g)	Calculated Oxalate per Serving
20 mg	1 medium tomatillo	34 g	7 mg

Remark: Low oxalate food (Less than 25 mg per serving)

Tomato

Avg Oxalate per 100 g	Serving Size	Serving (g)	Calculated Oxalate per Serving
9 mg	1 cup, sliced	180 g	17 mg

Remark: Low oxalate food (Less than 25 mg per serving).

Tomato Juice

Avg Oxalate per 100 g	Serving Size	Serving (g)	Calculated Oxalate per Serving
5 mg	1 cup	250 g	12 mg

Remark: Low oxalate food (Less than 25 mg per serving).

Tortilla (Corn or Flour)

Avg Oxalate per 100 g	Serving Size	Serving (g)	Calculated Oxalate per Serving
35 mg	1 medium	49 g	17 mg

Remark: Low oxalate food (Less than 25 mg per serving).

Tortilla Chips

Avg Oxalate per 100 g	Serving Size	Serving (g)	Calculated Oxalate per Serving
34 mg	1 oz	28 g	10 mg

Remark: Low oxalate food (Less than 25 mg per serving).

Turkey

Avg Oxalate per 100 g	Serving Size	Serving (g)	Calculated Oxalate per Serving
0 mg	3 oz	85 g	0 mg

Remark: Low oxalate food (Less than 25 mg per serving).

Turmeric

Avg Oxalate per 100 g	Serving Size	Serving (g)	Calculated Oxalate per Serving
2107 mg	1 tsp	2.2 g	46 mg

Remark: Moderate oxalate food (25–99 mg per serving).

Turnip

Avg Oxalate per 100 g	Serving Size	Serving (g)	Calculated Oxalate per Serving
7 mg	½ cup, chopped	72 g	5 mg

Remark: Low oxalate food (Less than 25 mg per serving).

Vanilla Extract

Avg Oxalate per 100 g	Serving Size	Serving (g)	Calculated Oxalate per Serving
17 mg	1 tsp	5 g	1 mg

Remark: Low oxalate food (Less than 25 mg per serving).

Vanilla Wafers

Avg Oxalate per 100 g	Serving Size	Serving (g)	Calculated Oxalate per Serving
25 mg	8 cookies	30 g	7 mg

Remark: Low oxalate food (Less than 25 mg per serving).

Vegetable and Seed Oil

Avg Oxalate per 100 g	Serving Size	Serving (g)	Calculated Oxalate per Serving
5 mg	1 tbsp	13.5 g	0 mg

Remark: Low oxalate food (Less than 25 mg per serving).

Vegetable Quinoa (Soup)

Avg Oxalate per 100 g	Serving Size	Serving (g)	Calculated Oxalate per Serving
13 mg	1 cup	241 g	31 mg

Remark: Moderate oxalate food (25–99 mg per serving).

Vegetable Soup

Avg Oxalate per 100 g	Serving Size	Serving (g)	Calculated Oxalate per Serving
7 mg	½ cup	126 g	9 mg

Remark: Low oxalate food (Less than 25 mg per serving).

Vinegar

Avg Oxalate per 100 g	Serving Size	Serving (g)	Calculated Oxalate per Serving
4 mg	1 tbsp	15 g	1 mg

Remark: Low oxalate food (Less than 25 mg per serving).

Walnuts

Avg Oxalate per 100 g	Serving Size	Serving (g)	Calculated Oxalate per Serving
62 mg	¼ cup	29 g	18 mg

Remark: Low oxalate food (Less than 25 mg per serving).

Water Chestnuts

Avg Oxalate per 100 g	Serving Size	Serving (g)	Calculated Oxalate per Serving
2 mg	½ cup	70 g	1 mg

Remark: Low oxalate food (Less than 25 mg per serving).

Watercress (Raw)

Avg Oxalate per 100 g	Serving Size	Serving (g)	Calculated Oxalate per Serving
8 mg	1 cup	58 g	4 mg

Remark: Low oxalate food (Less than 25 mg per serving).

Watermelon

Avg Oxalate per 100 g	Serving Size	Serving (g)	Calculated Oxalate per Serving
1 mg	1 cup, cubed	160 g	2 mg

Remark: Low oxalate food (Less than 25 mg per serving).

Watermelon Seeds

Avg Oxalate per 100 g	Serving Size	Serving (g)	Calculated Oxalate per Serving
0 mg	1 oz	28.35 g	0 mg

Remark: Low oxalate food (Less than 25 mg per serving).

Wattle Seed

Avg Oxalate per 100 g	Serving Size	Serving (g)	Calculated Oxalate per Serving
104 mg	2 tbsp	20 g	21 mg

Remark: Low oxalate food (Less than 25 mg per serving).

Weetabix (Cereal)

Avg Oxalate per 100 g	Serving Size	Serving (g)	Calculated Oxalate per Serving
90 mg	2 biscuits	35 g	31 mg

Remark: **Moderate oxalate food (**25–99 mg per serving).

Wheat Flour (Gluten)

Avg Oxalate per 100 g	Serving Size	Serving (g)	Calculated Oxalate per Serving
54 mg	¼ cup	36 g	19 mg

Remark: **Low oxalate food** (Less than 25 mg per serving).

Wheat Germ

Avg Oxalate per 100 g	Serving Size	Serving (g)	Calculated Oxalate per Serving
81 mg	¼ cup	30 g	24 mg

Remark: **Low oxalate food** (Less than 25 mg per serving).

Whipped Cream

Avg Oxalate per 100 g	Serving Size	Serving (g)	Calculated Oxalate per Serving
2 mg	1 tbsp	6 g	0 mg

Remark: Low oxalate food (Less than 25 mg per serving).

White Bread

Avg Oxalate per 100 g	Serving Size	Serving (g)	Calculated Oxalate per Serving
24 mg	1 slice	30 g	7 mg

Remark: Low oxalate food (Less than 25 mg per serving).

White Chocolate

Avg Oxalate per 100 g	Serving Size	Serving (g)	Calculated Oxalate per Serving
8 mg	1 oz	28 g	2 mg

Remark: Low oxalate food (Less than 25 mg per serving).

White Pepper (Ground)

Avg Oxalate per 100 g	Serving Size	Serving (g)	Calculated Oxalate per Serving
29 mg	1 tsp (ground)	2.1 g	1 mg

Remark: Low oxalate food (Less than 25 mg per serving).

White Rice Flour

Avg Oxalate per 100 g	Serving Size	Serving (g)	Calculated Oxalate per Serving
25 mg	¼ cup	39.5 g	10 mg

Remark: Low oxalate food (Less than 25 mg per serving).

Whole Oat Bread

Avg Oxalate per 100 g	Serving Size	Serving (g)	Calculated Oxalate per Serving
44 mg	1 slice	30 g	13 mg

Remark: Low oxalate food (Less than 25 mg per serving).

Whole Wheat Bread

Avg Oxalate per 100 g	Serving Size	Serving (g)	Calculated Oxalate per Serving
27 mg	1 slice	24 g	6 mg

Remark: Low oxalate food (Less than 25 mg per serving).

Worcestershire Sauce

Avg Oxalate per 100 g	Serving Size	Serving (g)	Calculated Oxalate per Serving
20 mg	1 tbsp	16.8 g	3 mg

Remark: Low oxalate food (Less than 25 mg per serving).

Xylitol

Avg Oxalate per 100 g	Serving Size	Serving (g)	Calculated Oxalate per Serving
4 mg	1 tsp	3.2 g	0 mg

Remark: Low oxalate food (Less than 25 mg per serving).

Yam

Avg Oxalate per 100 g	Serving Size	Serving (g)	Calculated Oxalate per Serving
68 mg	½ cup	100 g	68 mg

Remark: **Moderate oxalate food** (25–99 mg per serving).

Yeast

Avg Oxalate per 100 g	Serving Size	Serving (g)	Calculated Oxalate per Serving
56 mg	1 tbsp	12.3 g	7 mg

Remark: **Low oxalate food** (Less than 25 mg per serving).

Yogurt (with Coconut)

Avg Oxalate per 100 g	Serving Size	Serving (g)	Calculated Oxalate per Serving
1 mg	6 oz	170 g	2 mg

Remark: **Low oxalate food** (Less than 25 mg per serving).

Yogurt (with Oat)

Avg Oxalate per 100 g	Serving Size	Serving (g)	Calculated Oxalate per Serving
2 mg	6 oz	170 g	3 mg

Remark: Low oxalate food (Less than 25 mg per serving).

Yogurt (with Soy)

Avg Oxalate per 100 g	Serving Size	Serving (g)	Calculated Oxalate per Serving
3 mg	6 oz	170 g	5 mg

Remark: Low oxalate food (Less than 25 mg per serving).

Zucchini

Avg Oxalate per 100 g	Serving Size	Serving (g)	Calculated Oxalate per Serving
6 mg	1 cup, chopped	124 g	7 mg

Remark: Low oxalate food (Less than 25 mg per serving).